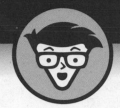

P9-DMX-629

Keto Diet

by Rami Abrams and Vicky Abrams

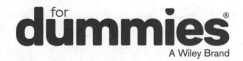

for
dummies®
A Wiley Brand

Keto Diet For Dummies®

Published by: **John Wiley & Sons, Inc.**, 111 River Street, Hoboken, NJ 07030-5774, www.wiley.com

Copyright © 2019 by John Wiley & Sons, Inc., Hoboken, New Jersey

Published simultaneously in Canada

For general information on our other products and services, please contact our Customer Care Department within the U.S. at 877-762-2974, outside the U.S. at 317-572-3993, or fax 317-572-4002. For technical support, please visit https://hub.wiley.com/community/support/dummies.

Wiley publishes in a variety of print and electronic formats and by print-on-demand. Some material included with standard print versions of this book may not be included in e-books or in print-on-demand. If this book refers to media such as a CD or DVD that is not included in the version you purchased, you may download this material at http://booksupport.wiley.com. For more information about Wiley products, visit www.wiley.com.

Library of Congress Control Number: 2019943091

ISBN 978-1-119-57892-5 (pbk); ISBN 978-1-119-57893-2 (ebk); ISBN 978-1-119-57940-3 (ebk)

Manufactured in the United States of America

SKY10030560_101421

Contents at a Glance

Recipes at a Glance

Side Dishes

Desserts

Table of Contents

Introduction

Are you interested in dropping a significant amount of weight in a relatively short period of time? Tired of crash diets that restrict your calories to near-starvation levels, only to have the weight rush back with a vengeance when you return to eating normally? Has your doctor told you to lower your cholesterol or watch your blood sugar? It may surprise you to know that you can achieve all your weight loss goals by changing what and how you eat. The standard American diet (appropriately abbreviated as SAD) is based around consuming extremely high levels of carbohydrates and minimizing the amount of fat you ingest. Although it's certainly possible to live this way, as humans have been doing since the agricultural revolution, it isn't actually the best way to live. A much better approach to eating focuses on low amounts of carbohydrates and high levels of fat — this approach is known as the *ketogenic diet* (or keto for short).

With all these advantages that have been repeatedly validated by peer-reviewed scientific studies, you may wonder why anyone would ever say anything negative about keto. Unfortunately, there is some reason for criticism. The primary issue most people have with the diet is more psychological than anything: Humans seem almost predisposed to look for "miracle cures," "superfoods," and anything else that seems too good to be true. As the saying goes, anything that seems too good to be true probably is. Keto isn't magic. It is, however, a completely natural metabolic process that's been ignored for most of civilized human history — not because carbohydrates are better for us, but because of how easily accessible they've been. Our society has become a chronic over-consumer of carbs and a systemic under-consumer of fats, leading to medical conditions that are simply the inevitable result of an imbalanced way of eating. Keto corrects this and does so in such a drastic manner that it can seem miraculous at times. If anything, however, these rapid and seemingly overwhelming benefits are more indicative of how imbalanced our eating patterns have become than they are of the "miracle" of keto.

Another legitimate source of criticism revolves around people who are always looking for a quick fix for anything. We guarantee that you interact with individuals like this regularly — people who constantly have the right answer, who can tell you one quick fix to completely resolve any problem area in your life, and who seem to oversimplify virtually everything. It's an unfortunate reality that many people with this mind-set have jumped on the keto bandwagon, and the diet has garnered a lot of negative attention as a result. However, it's important not to throw the baby out with the bathwater — just because some low-carb advocates have the wrong mind-set toward the diet doesn't mean that this nutritional approach is without merit.

We freely acknowledge that "crash" or "fad" diets are unhealthy. Even if they seem to work in the short term, that weight always comes roaring back with a vengeance the moment you resume normal eating patterns. We're huge advocates of maintaining a healthy lifestyle that's nutritious, delicious, and comfortable. For us, keto isn't a short-term quick fix for anything — it's the way we live, and you couldn't pay us to go back.

Weight loss is the most high-profile benefit of keto, particularly in today's environment of unhealthy eating and equally unrealistic body image expectations. However, it isn't the primary reason we've adhered to a ketogenic lifestyle for years. When you maintain a diet that's filled with healthy, satiating fats, your energy levels and mental clarity remain steady and unobstructed throughout the day. Our focus is sharper, we don't experience the highs and lows of blood sugar spikes, and it's been years since we felt "hangry."

What you won't find in this book is an encouragement to change your eating habits for a short period to experience rapid weight loss. Although it's common for people on keto to burn through fat rapidly, this isn't a crash diet you should go on for two weeks before a wedding, and then transition right back to high-carb eating. We highly recommend that you consider making a lifestyle change to a much healthier diet that has numerous proven benefits. You don't need to decide to do keto forever at this point, but we'd be surprised if you aren't strongly considering it after a month on healthy fats — you'll look and feel that good.

About This Book

We've written this book so you can find information quickly and easily. Each chapter focuses on a specific aspect of the ketogenic diet and outlines how to make the transition, accentuating benefits or minimizing downsides, and structuring your diet and lifestyle to create your best "you." There are quite a few specific details and practical tips, but you don't have to read the book from front to back. Feel free to skip around, browse the sections that you find interesting, and just follow where your questions take you.

Reading this entire book isn't necessary to experience a successful keto journey. We've designed it as a resource you can refer to continually. Make notes in the margins, jot down additional resources or recipe adjustments, and highlight information you find most applicable to your unique situation. In short, make this book a reflection of your ketogenic exploration, and customize it to fit you!

Throughout the book you'll notice text marked by the Technical Stuff icon, as well as sidebars (text in gray boxes). If you're short on time, you can skip both of these kinds of text — they're interesting, but not essential to understanding the topic at hand.

Finally, within this book, you may note that some web addresses break across two lines of text. If you're reading this book in print and want to visit one of these web pages, simply key in the web address exactly as it's noted in the text, pretending as though the line break doesn't exist. If you're reading this as an e-book, you've got it easy — just click the web address to be taken directly to the web page.

Foolish Assumptions

As we wrote this book, we made the following assumptions about you:

>> You want to change your diet, lose weight, improve your fitness, or manage some type of medical condition.

>> You have control over your and your family's food choices, and you want to encourage your family to enjoy a healthy, low-carb lifestyle.

>> You want to minimize processed and unhealthy junk foods and maximize wholesome food choices to feel younger, healthier, and happier.

>> You're interested in learning how food choices affect you physically and mentally, but you don't want to get bogged down in all the scientific jargon. You want a summary of what you need to know in plain English.

>> You're open to the idea of making lifestyle changes — avoiding certain foods, making sleep a priority, adopting a fitness program — to enhance your quality of life.

Icons Used in This Book

Throughout this book, we use *icons* (little pictures in the margin) to draw your attention to certain kinds of information. Here are the icons we use, and what they mean:

TIP

Whenever you see the Tip icon, you can be sure to find a nugget of information that will make your life on keto easier in some way, big or small.

REMEMBER

This book is a reference, which means you don't have to commit it to memory and there won't be a test on Friday. However, sometimes we do tell you something that's so important that you'll want to file it away for future use, and when we do, we mark that information with the Remember icon.

WARNING

When you see the Warning icon, beware! We're letting you know about a pitfall or danger that you'll want to avoid.

TECHNICAL STUFF

Sometimes we wade into the weeds and tell you something super-technical or scientific. This is the kind of stuff we thrive on, but if you're not as geeky as we are, you can skip this without missing anything essential.

Finally, we use a little tomato icon (🍅) to highlight vegetarian recipes in the Recipes in This Chapter lists, as well as in the Recipes at a Glance at the front of this book.

Beyond the Book

In addition to the book you have in your hand, you can access some helpful extra content online. Check out the free Cheat Sheet Keto Diet For Dummies. You can access it by going to www.dummies.com and entering **Keto Diet For Dummies** in the Search box.

Where to Go from Here

You can read this book from beginning to end, or you can use the table of contents and index to locate the topics you're most interested in right now. If you're not sure where to start, you can't go wrong with Chapter 1. If you'd rather start cooking, head to Part 5, or use the Recipes at a Glance at the start of the book to find the kind of recipe you're looking for, from appetizers to desserts. If you're curious about fasting, Chapter 12 is for you. And if you'd just like a quick reminder of ten great benefits of being in ketosis, head to Chapter 21. Wherever you start, we hope the keto diet is as rewarding for you as it is for us!

1

Getting Started with the Keto Diet

Get acquainted with the foundations of keto.

Identify the positives and negatives of low-carb living.

Understand the science behind the keto diet.

Discover the keto building blocks.

Chapter **1**

Brushing Up on the Basics

K eto has become quite popular over the past several years, but what do you really know about this seemingly trendy dietary lifestyle? Is keto truly worth the hype, and is it really a healthy way to lose weight? We're here to help you figure out if keto is right for you and the basic steps of following a keto lifestyle safely and effectively. In this chapter, we cover the nuts and bolts of the keto lifestyle and get you ready to go, with a clear sense of the benefits of making a keto choice.

Understanding What the Keto Diet Is

The ketogenic diet (or keto diet for short) is an exceptionally well-researched and proven method to start working *with* your body, rather than against it, to improve your health. Following the basic rules of the keto lifestyle can help you

» Feel more energized.

» Lose weight faster.

» Improve the health of your heart.

» Sharpen your mental focus.

In addition to these benefits, there are a host of other long-term benefits that will leave you jumping for joy. Though it's become popular recently, the keto diet has been used for almost a hundred years to heal and prevent disease — that's a long track record of benefits.

In a nutshell, the keto diet is

>> High fat

>> Moderate protein

>> Very low carbohydrate

Having grains and carbohydrates form the basis of every meal may seem like contemporary wisdom, but for most of human history, this wasn't the case. Processed and easily digested carbohydrates fuel weight gain and unhealthy spikes in blood sugar with each bite; over the course of a lifetime, this destroys your health.

The keto diet puts your body into *ketosis,* a process where you use fats, rather than sugars from carbohydrates, to fuel your body. On the keto diet, you learn to turn nutritional powerhouses — fats — into the basis of your meals.

In this chapter, and again in Chapter 3, we allay the fears that are commonly encountered when we talk about eating fat. The truth is that fat really isn't to blame for the increasingly common problems of obesity and being overweight that you always hear about. Fat is actually very good for you, keeps you feeling fuller longer, helps you lose weight, and improves your health over the long term.

There are a lot of misconceptions about nutrition in general, and the keto diet in particular. In this book, we wade through the incessant chatter about what you should and shouldn't eat to get to the meat of it all (pun intended). The keto lifestyle is much more than the "bacon wrapped in cheese" memes will have you believe — although you can eat cheese and bacon. It won't wreak havoc on your heart or blood vessels, nor will it increase your cholesterol levels if you follow a whole-food-based keto lifestyle.

Despite what many of us have been told for decades, we don't need to eat many carbohydrates as part of a healthy lifestyle. Instead, eating a range of whole keto foods can be the key to healthy living. Keto is a flexible and adventurous lifestyle that isn't a one-size-fits-all plan; there are several different varieties to fit with your lifestyle and goals.

In the following sections, we look at the various options available, how they're different, and what each has to offer.

THE HISTORY OF KETO

The ketogenic diet has been around in one form or another for thousands of years; in fact, the first mention of this way of eating was found in Greek medical texts from 400 B.C. The diet was formally created and named a century ago by medical doctors who were seeking an innovative way to treat epilepsy in children. It was very successful, although the medical community didn't completely understand *how* it worked — they simply knew that consuming a high-fat, low-carbohydrate diet drastically reduced, and occasionally even eliminated, the number of seizures epileptic patients experienced.

The diet became less popular in the 1930s and 1940s as antiseizure drugs were invented. The primary selling point for these medications was their convenience, not necessarily their effectiveness. Keto is still so effective that it's nearly always what doctors turn to in cases of *intractable epilepsy,* a version of the condition that is unaffected by medication. In these cases, keto nearly always works. The primary objection to the diet, and why it fell out of favor in the 1930s and 1940s, is that it requires quite a bit of dedication and discipline to cook in a way that's completely different from the way the rest of society approaches food. The benefits are undeniable, but it does take effort — and if you can treat epilepsy by simply popping a pill, that's a much more convenient approach than totally revamping your diet. For the approximately 30 percent of epileptic patients for whom medication has no effect, however, keto offers much-needed relief.

Between the 1940s and the 1990s, the ketogenic diet fell into some level of obscurity. It was still used in the medical community, but sparingly, and it didn't generate a tremendous amount of discussion. That changed in the mid-1990s when Hollywood director Jim Abrahams discovered the diet as he desperately searched for treatments that would help his epileptic son. The Abrahams found keto to be so effective that Jim created the Charlie Foundation, named after his child, to bring the eating approach back as a mainstream treatment. Abrahams's efforts marked a resurgence of interest in ketosis, and over the next several decades, thousands of studies were conducted on the ketogenic diet by the medical and scientific community.

As the diet's resurgence continued, people began to notice that it had uses beyond preventing seizures. In the early 1900s, the prevalence of diabetes was roughly 3 in 100,000; a hundred years later, however, nearly 1 in 10 Americans are diabetic or prediabetic. Those who began trying ketosis were shocked by the results: Not only did it help more than 90 percent of type 2 diabetics reduce their medication, but more than half of type 2 diabetics who stuck with the low-carb, high-fat lifestyle experienced such an incredible reduction in their HbA1C levels (the primary marker of diabetes) that their condition was effectively reversed!

(continued)

(continued)

The diabetic community reacted with understandable excitement, and people began to notice other effects. Individuals who stayed on the ketogenic diet watched excess pounds melt away, and they naturally assumed a healthy body weight, regardless of age, gender, race, or ethnicity — it didn't even seem to matter if someone exercised or not. Keto was conducive to maintaining ideal body fat percentages.

Weight loss is a multibillion-dollar industry, so this discovery spurred a tremendous amount of interest. New research began to discover that this way of eating lowered low-density lipoprotein (LDL) cholesterol (the bad kind) and raised high-density lipoprotein (HDL) cholesterol (the good kind), which completely shocked the diet community of the 1990s. Women who suffered from polycystic ovary syndrome (PCOS) experienced a reduction in symptoms, and studies confirmed that aspiring mothers who struggled with fertility issues had statistically significant improved rates of conception while eating low-carb.

Stories of people beating cancer with keto began to surface, and, as you can imagine, this generated quite the buzz in the medical community. Studies found that keto wasn't a cure for cancer, but it did have several remarkable effects. The first was that many cancerous tumors feed almost exclusively on glucose but can't be fueled by ketones; when patients transitioned to a different way of eating, even some aggressive forms of cancer stopped growing, giving traditional medical treatments more time to work. Studies also confirmed that a ketogenic lifestyle made tumors more sensitive to radiation and chemotherapy — not only did the diet give the medical community more time to work, but it actually assisted their efforts.

Standard ketogenic diet

The standard ketogenic diet is the basic version of the keto diet. It's been around the longest and has the most evidence and research behind it. If you're thinking about keto, you need to be very familiar with the standard ketogenic diet. It clearly breaks down the sources of your daily calorie intake, as follows:

>> **Fat:** 70 percent

>> **Protein:** 25 percent

>> **Carbohydrates:** 5 percent

Historically, on this diet, you'll generally eat about 25 grams of carbohydrates per day. However, we live in more flexible times, and some people eat as much as 50 grams per day. That's okay, because most people stay in ketosis on 50 grams of carbs a day, so they don't need to limit their carbs anymore. Over time, you'll figure out what works best for you.

The amount of daily carbs is, at most, only a fifth of what many Americans eat. On the standard American diet, you get about 30 percent of calories from fat, 20 percent from protein, and 50 percent (or more) from carbohydrates. That means most Americans are eating about 250 grams of carbs or more per day. As you can imagine, making such a radical change from a carb-based diet to a fat-based one will have a massive impact on your health and energy levels.

On the standard ketogenic diet, the ratio is 70:25:5 in terms of calories coming from fat, protein, and carbs. You should aim for 30 grams of carbs or fewer in a day.

REMEMBER

Targeted ketogenic diet

The targeted ketogenic diet is geared toward athletes. It's a slightly more flexible version of the keto diet because it allows you to eat more carbs around the time of your intense workouts. When you're burning a lot of calories, the carbs you eat are consumed as fuel immediately, so your body doesn't get "kicked out" of ketosis in the long term. As soon as you use up all the carbs during your workout, your body goes back to fat burning because there aren't carbs left around when you're more sedentary.

This choice is good for very active people who are exercising at high levels regularly (for hours, not minutes) or training for an intense athletic challenge that requires a lot of energy, like a marathon. Regardless, this is not a free pass to eat as many carbohydrates as you would on a high-carb diet. You should consume about 20 or 25 grams of easily digestible carbs approximately 30 to 45 minutes before you exercise. After exercising, you'll go back to the regular keto diet. Keep in mind the total number of calories (including your pre-workout carbs) when coming up with your daily energy intake.

It's critical that you only eat enough carbs to fuel your workout, so your body goes back to burning fats when you're done exercising. Generally, you should be well adjusted to the standard ketogenic diet for a couple months at least before you switch to this targeted version.

REMEMBER

Cyclical ketogenic diet

The cyclical ketogenic diet is another more flexible keto option for highly trained athletes. We're upping the playing field here — this is the ultramarathon runner or the professional athlete, not the weekend warrior. These athletes may increase their carb intake for a short time to "fuel" themselves for the high level of performance they're about to commit to. The increase may be for a couple of days before a major training event — and the amount of carbs they consume is in line with the amount of physical activity they're facing. Then they go back to the standard ketogenic diet after the major event is over. Although they may be out of ketosis during these "cheat days," their high level of performance ensures that they're still in the low-carb range because they're burning so many more calories than usual.

Another group of people who follow the cyclical ketogenic diet are those who have a hard time sticking to the standard ketogenic diet and choose to have cheat days once in a while. This may involve going keto five days a week, with the weekends reserved for "cheat days." For those who eat carbs on the weekend, or can't stick to the standard ketogenic diet because of social pressures, it's important not to go on carb-binging cycles. It's quite a shift for the body to go from ketosis to high-carb so rapidly. Instead, increase your carbs to a "low-carb diet," in the range of 150 to 200 grams on your cheat days. You won't be in ketosis on those days — and it may take a while for your body to go back to ketosis even on your regular standard ketogenic diet days — but at least you'll still have the benefits of cutting back on carbs.

TIP

The cyclical ketogenic diet may be helpful for athletes and those who find it difficult to commit to the keto lifestyle. Keto is very flexible and can work with any lifestyle, as long as you make a commitment to health.

High-protein ketogenic diet

In the high-protein ketogenic diet, you increase the percent of calories from protein. Commonly, this breaks down as follows:

» **Fat:** 60 percent

» **Protein:** 35 percent

» **Carbohydrate:** 5 percent

This option is best for people who are concerned about losing muscle or even want to bulk up, like bodybuilders or individuals who have very low lean body muscle mass. Generally, keto is a muscle neutral diet (you don't gain or lose it), so adding protein is a great choice for those who want to gain muscle. In this diet, you're still in ketosis, but you don't necessarily have as high a level of ketones as someone on the standard ketogenic diet. It's hard, but possible, to get kicked out of ketosis if you go higher than the recommended 35 percent of calories from protein. It's also important on this type of keto diet to remember to eat a range of protein foods that are healthy and nutritious.

Deciding Whether the Keto Diet Is Right for You

Still unsure if the keto diet is right for you? In addition to the four options we just looked at, the keto lifestyle can be adapted to fit almost everyone's needs — from the person seeking to jump-start weight loss to the person concerned about risk of diabetes. It does take a can-do attitude and commitment because you'll encounter some bumps in the road, but for those who press on, the keto lifestyle is well worth the effort. We dive more into the many benefits — and few side effects — of the keto lifestyle in Chapter 2, but in this section we give you a little taste of why the keto diet may be right for you.

You want to lose weight fast and keep it off

If you've tried multiple diets and feel discouraged because you can't keep the weight off, the keto diet is for you. Keto turns your body into a fat-burning machine. With the right blend of exercise and a well-balanced keto diet, you can reach your weight-loss goals. The keto diet has been shown to help people lose weight faster than low-fat diets; if you stay committed, it's a healthy and satisfying way to maintain your weight over the long term.

You're not afraid of a little commitment

Keto is great for those who can commit to it. There is some built-in flexibility to keto, but changing your mind-set to a "fat is healthy, and carbs aren't as necessary as we thought" mentality requires some nutritional know-how (reading this book is a great start) and a commitment to choosing keto-friendly options in a sea of high-carb treats. You need to make some thoughtful choices about what you put into your body as fuel — looking at your long-term goals, rather than what is readily available.

You may find this challenging, especially in the first few days and weeks, if you notice some tell-tale signs of the *keto flu* (the muscle cramping and general feeling of being run down as your body adjusts to ketosis). We share some tips to decrease or avoid the symptoms in Chapter 3, but going through the keto flu may make you doubt your commitment to the keto lifestyle. If you're serious about your health and you aren't easily swayed by a few bumps along the way, keto offers lasting benefits.

You want to decrease your risk of diabetes

If you're concerned about your risk of getting diabetes, keto is an excellent option for you. Eating a keto diet stops the wild up and down sugar spikes associated with the standard American diet, which is loaded with carbohydrates. Keto can help reduce your risk of getting type 2 diabetes — a widespread problem that leads to heart disease and other major medical issues. Alarmingly, up to one-third of Americans are prediabetic and don't even know it.

WARNING

Be cautious, however, if you are diabetic. Research is showing that the keto diet may actually help cure diabetes and get people off medications, but diabetes can be a severe medical condition that requires a doctor's care. It's best to have the support of a doctor or nutritionist if you're already diagnosed with diabetes and you want to try the keto diet. It can lower your blood sugar levels too much if you're already taking certain medications.

You're tired of feeling run down and sluggish

Most people on the keto diet realize they have more energy and mental focus. We've almost forgotten what it feels like to have the "hangry" feeling we used to get around 4 p.m. — when we'd feel justified for biting off a coworker's head if we couldn't eat something, anything, right that minute.

These symptoms are practically universal when your body relies on the wild swings in blood sugar level that happen when you eat carbohydrates but haven't had a meal in several hours. The keto diet allows you to break free from these symptoms because your blood glucose levels stay stable, whether you're in the middle of a meal or you haven't had a bite to eat in over six hours. With stable blood sugar levels, you're energized and don't feel a sluggish at the end of the day — or at any other time.

You want to get healthy and stay that way for a long time

The keto diet is not just good for weight loss and sugar control; it's also an anti-inflammatory diet that can improve your health in many other areas as well. The diet was initially developed for children with incurable seizures who weren't getting better, despite having access to the newest and best medicines.

The keto diet was able to decrease, and often completely stop, their seizures. Subsequent research suggests that the keto diet helps reduce the risk of neurodegenerative diseases like Alzheimer's disease, can work to improve your cholesterol levels, and may prevent heart disease. A bonus for teenagers is that it may even be a treatment if you're acne prone. We get into the details of the many health benefits of the keto diet in later chapters, but we can let you know now, there are quite a few.

REMEMBER

The keto diet may be for you if you're ready to make the commitment to changing your health for the better.

Flipping the Switch on Your Metabolism

Getting into ketosis requires a commitment to drastically cutting your carbohydrate intake. Your body is geared to using carbohydrates as fuel if they're available, so you won't go into ketosis until you drop to 50 grams or fewer of carbohydrates a day and maintain that level of carb intake for at least several days. If you go back to eating more carbs, you'll be kicked out of ketosis. Learning how to get into ketosis is vital to enjoying a keto lifestyle. We're here to help you figure it all out.

Consuming the right ratio of macronutrients: Fat, protein, and carbs

When you start a keto diet, you'll need to be very clear on the number of calories you're getting from the three primary *macronutrients* (the main groups of food that provide fuel for your body): fats, protein, and carbs. The key to keto is that you're getting only a small amount of your nutrition from carbs. Even if you eat a high-fat and moderate-protein diet, if you go over your carb limit, you'll be kicked out of ketosis. You'll have to monitor your carb intake closely until you get used to being on a very low-carb diet and have a good sense of the amount of carbs in different foods. This will mean understanding the ratio of macros in a serving size when you eat fresh foods and always, always checking the nutrition labels when you eat anything from a package.

As you start looking more closely at nutrition labels, you'll be surprised at how many foods have hidden carbs, from condiments like ketchup and salad dressing to meats and other proteins that have flour or breading added. You'll also have to keep this inquisitive nature up when you go out to eat, even if it's at a friend's house. Being aware of what goes into your food is your number-one priority.

Upping your consumption of healthy fats

As you know, you'll need to increase your fat intake — and by a lot. If you've ever been on a diet, it can be quite alarming to have to raise your fat intake, especially if you think eating fat will automatically make you fat. Even if you're not looking to lose any weight, fat has received a reputation for being unhealthy, bad for your heart, and something that should always be limited. This couldn't be further from the truth. Of course, you'll want to make sure you get fat from healthy sources and choose a range of nutritious fats, but fats themselves aren't inherently bad. We talk more about this in Chapter 4, but it's important that you're getting your fats from both plant and animal foods and eating a mix of nuts and seeds, avocados, healthy oils, dairy, and animal fat.

Calculating your protein target

The amount of protein you get in a keto diet isn't that far off from what you'd eat on a high-carb diet, so there shouldn't be too much confusion here. Some people wrongly think that the keto diet is a high-protein diet and that all people on the diet eat is meat, meat, and more meat. This isn't true, and the keto diet isn't an excuse to only eat beef jerky and hamburger patties. You'll need to be aware of how much protein you should be consuming in a day based on your body weight and activity level. You'll also need to get familiar with the appropriate serving sizes of your protein sources, as well as the best sources of protein that work with your lifestyle. A moderate amount of protein is about 0.36 gram for every pound of body weight if you're usually sedentary, or about 54 grams if you weigh 150 pounds.

Slashing your carb intake

Your carb intake will make or break your keto journey, so be vigilant! We should mention that whenever we talk about "carbs" in this book, we're referring to digestible carbs. These are complex and simple carbohydrates — from whole grains and oatmeal to candy and sugar-sweetened anything — that your body uses as fuel. You don't have to limit indigestible carbohydrates like fiber; your body can't digest them, which means carbs from fiber won't kick you out of ketosis. In the keto diet, you exchange high-carb foods for low-carb vegetables that are also good sources of fiber. You can eat a small amount of low-sugar fruits like berries. Don't worry, there are lots of great-tasting low-carb options that will keep you full.

To succeed on the keto diet, get used to looking at nutrition labels. It's important for you to know how many carbs you're eating so you don't get kicked out of ketosis. Over time, you'll learn how to avoid "hidden" carbs and thrive on low-carb options instead.

Knowing when you've entered a state of ketosis

It takes between a few days to a week of a very low-carb diet before most people enter ketosis. That's because our bodies store an "emergency" amount of carbs just in case we suddenly run out of bread and pasta. If it's your first time entering ketosis, you may be unsure of what to expect. Some people have symptoms that suggest ketosis, while others won't notice any changes at all. The most common signs of ketosis for first-timers are headaches, fatigue, and muscle cramps (symptoms of the keto flu that we cover in Chapter 2). Although unpleasant, this is a sign that you're achieving your goal.

So, how will you know you're in ketosis if you don't have any symptoms? One common way to tell if you're in ketosis is to use a ketosis urine test — it's the same concept as the urine test women use to check if they're pregnant, but instead you'll find out if you've succeeded into getting into ketosis. When you're in ketosis, your urine will have a certain level of *ketones* (the products of fatty acids breaking down) that high-carb dieters won't. This lets you know that you've reached your goal. These urine sticks are available online or at most quality nutrition stores. You can also take a blood test to measure the same thing. We show you exactly how to test for ketosis in Chapter 3.

Knowing when to stop

When you're clearly in ketosis and you've gotten over any initial roadblocks, you should be feeling on top of the world. Occasionally, though, some people in ketosis don't feel this way even after weeks or months of commitment. Here are some signs that you need to reevaluate your approach to keto:

>> You're constantly tired.

>> It's difficult to get a good night's sleep.

>> Your bathroom habits have slowed way down.

>> You're not as strong as you used to be and you've lost muscle definition.

>> You're experiencing skin rashes or hair loss.

If you're dealing with some of these issues, you probably need to make a change and investigate what's going wrong with your keto journey. You may notice these side effects if you aren't following a whole foods diet and are missing out on crucial nutrients, like essential vitamins and minerals. Some of us fall into this trap because we eat the same five or six keto-friendly foods and not much else. If you feel like you're floundering in your keto diet, make sure you take stock of what you eat on a daily basis and if it's genuinely nurturing you.

WARNING

A rare side effect, but one that deserves mention, is *ketoacidosis.* This most often occurs in type 1 diabetics, but it can occasionally be experienced by others. Ketoacidosis is when the number of ketones in your bloodstream have exceeded the healthy range. This generally only occurs in people who have an underlying medical condition (like diabetes), but very rarely it can happen if you follow ketosis and restrict your calories too much or have a high energy requirement, like women who are pregnant. If you have a significant medical condition, talk with your doctor before starting a keto diet.

TIP

If you have a medical condition that you manage with a doctor, make sure to seek your doctor's advice before starting keto. Keto is a healthy lifestyle option, but some medical conditions don't mix well with it.

Clearing Common Hurdles

The keto diet can be challenging at first, so you need to focus on your commitment before beginning the journey. It's a good idea to have a sense of the common hurdles you'll likely encounter when you start the keto diet so you can be prepared to face them confidently. We get into the nuts and bolts of this in Chapter 3, but here we give you a little taste of what to expect.

We've found it's a good idea to have clear and specific reasons to start the keto lifestyle. "Losing weight" or "getting healthy" are common reasons people begin dieting, but to succeed at such a significant switch, you need to dig deeper and find the reasons that are unique to you. These reasons will motivate you when you have a carb craving or feel like you just don't have anything to eat. For some people, it's losing weight to run the marathon on their bucket list; for others, it's getting healthy so they don't end up with diabetes like their parents.

TIP

Whatever your reason, write it down — and have it readily available — so that when you encounter hurdles, you remember why you started in the first place. When you have concrete goals and a specific plan to accomplish them, you'll be more likely to find success in your journey.

Another great idea is getting an accountability partner, someone you trust and who will hold you accountable. Make sure it's someone you talk with or see regularly so he can check in on you and keep you motivated.

REMEMBER

Like anything that's worth it, you'll come across a few hurdles as you transition into keto. Being prepared and having a plan are essential to maintaining the keto lifestyle.

Dietary restrictions

The first thing that people get concerned about are the restrictions of the keto lifestyle. Because so many of us consume half (or more!) of our calories in the form of carbohydrates, you may feel like you have nothing to eat. This couldn't be further from the truth. There is quite a range of high-fat, low-carbohydrate foods out there that you haven't explored. The keto lifestyle will open up a world of healthy whole foods that will keep you satisfied and healthy.

Carb cravings

Giving up something always leaves intense cravings until the void is filled. Carbs are no different. It's normal to have intense cravings for carbs when you first go on the keto diet, especially because your body is so used to using them as fuel. What's more, you're probably a bit addicted to carbs. Sugar triggers the same receptors in your brain as heroin, so when you give up carbs, you're literally giving up an addiction.

Luckily, there is also a range of alternative "flours" and low-carb snacks that you can have on hand as you start the keto lifestyle. With a little knowledge and some trial and error, you'll beat the carb cravings and find foods you enjoy that keep you satisfied without intense cravings. As you get further into the keto lifestyle, however, you'll realize that your cravings for carbs will disappear altogether. You'll lose the urge to snack between meals as your glucose levels stabilize and you feel satisfied with your whole-food keto meals.

Unpleasant side effects

Keto can be associated with unpleasant side effects that you just have to get through. Keto flu and *keto breath* (the fruitlike and sometimes musty mouth odor that happens during ketosis) are just some of the hurdles you'll get familiar with during your keto journey. These are a double-edged sword: They mean that you're getting into ketosis, which is the goal, but they can still be challenging to navigate. Some people notice constipation or may even have nutritional deficiencies as they try to figure out what to eat on a regular basis. These are the growing pains of ketosis, and they work themselves out if you're patient and you persevere. This book gives you the tools to make your transition easier and limit the side effects, but you'll have to bring the commitment and drive to see it through.

Social pressures

Eating is quite the social event, and many people will have an opinion about what you should and shouldn't eat. People unfamiliar with the keto lifestyle will worry that you'll end up having a heart attack or other health problems; these concerns are completely unfounded or are based on misconceptions. If you've done your research and you're committed to your path, don't let their worries or even fears get you off track. You know what's best for your body and how to fuel it better than even your well-meaning friends, family, or coworkers. Thank them for their concern and let them know you've done your research and you're committed. When they begin to see the results of keto, they may change their tune. You may even be able to teach them a thing or two about nutrition.

Restaurants, family gatherings, and parties may be challenging as you transition to keto: You'll have to navigate breads, desserts, and other high-carb treats. People will naturally be curious if they notice that you're staying away from certain foods, and they may want to give you their opinions. Don't get hung up on whether they agree.

Another social pressure you may encounter is one from your doctor. Physicians are trained to go with long-established science and tend to be wary of "new" ways of approaching health. Keto has a long and well-established medical history, but a lot of that history revolved around treating patients for epilepsy. If you told your doctor that you were on keto to prevent seizures, he likely wouldn't bat an eye. But if you mention that you're doing it to treat another condition (like diabetes or high cholesterol), he may be a bit more reluctant to give you his blessing. Have a frank discussion with him about the research you've done, specifically referring him to many of the peer-reviewed medical and scientific studies we frequently reference on our websites (www.tasteaholics.com and www.sonourished.com).

You can also try to suggest a monitored approach where your visit your doctor every few months for a checkup and blood test. This method would provide you with measurable results and will build confidence in both you and your doctor.

You know your body best, and if you've done your research, stay empowered to care for your body in the way that makes you feel at your best.

Don't let well-meaning friends, family, or even doctors dissuade you from pursuing a healthy whole-foods keto lifestyle. Keep committed and keep doing what's right for your lifestyle and healthy body.

Chapter 2

Weighing the Pros and Cons of the Keto Diet

The ketogenic diet is not only an intuitive and simple way to eat, but also a lifestyle choice proven to improve your health and keep you feeling your best. Eating the nutritious, high-quality foods found on the keto diet fuels you with clean energy, letting your mind and body do what comes naturally: Be strong and efficient, prevent disease, and maintain a clear and optimistic outlook on life.

Sadly, many people have fallen away from this way of eating and coming back to it may seem overwhelming at first, especially if you're a bit rusty on the topics of ketosis, macros, and metabolism. There's no need to worry, though. In this book, we guide you through the basics, and this foundation will help you breeze through many of the misunderstandings that you'll encounter on your keto journey. With a little thoughtfulness and persistence, you'll soon notice the many benefits of the keto diet, and these concerns will drop away.

In this chapter, we discuss the main benefits of keto — get ready, because it's not a short list! We also walk you through some of the common concerns people have when starting a keto diet, especially in the first few days and weeks. We dive into the common misconception that a high-fat diet will make you fat or unhealthy (spoiler alert: it won't). Instead, we point out the real culprits — sugar and processed foods — and show you how life without them can be so much sweeter.

The Numerous Benefits of a Keto Diet

You may not know it, but the keto diet is not just a fad. The keto diet uses fat as fuel to steer the body into *ketogenesis,* a process that pushes the body to use more effective ways to energize and heal itself. Since the medical community began formally using the ketogenic diet as a treatment back in the 1920s, doctors and scientists have been aware of ketones' ability to heal the body of debilitating conditions that modern medicine gave up on as untreatable, like refractory epilepsy. Since the 1920s, the keto diet has provided many more benefits than just treating epilepsy — everything from weight loss to improved cardiovascular health. When you recognize these benefits, you'll be eager to hop on the keto diet bandwagon.

Weight loss

Let's address the elephant in the room head-on: Fat does not make you fat. The human body is much more intricate and intuitive than that. The idea that "fat makes you fat" is a gimmick used by corporate interests that have fueled the high-sugar, low-fat diet craze of the 1980s and 1990s, which only managed to make many of us fatter, sicker, and addicted to sugar. The number of people who struggle with obesity has doubled since that era, while the ketogenic diet has been used since the 1960s to stop excessive weight gain in its tracks.

Using fat as fuel bypasses sugar's addictive chemistry and ensures that we use those pesky love handles and muffin tops that we already have as our source of energy. Because the body has an infinite ability to store fat (compared to the much more limited ability to store carbohydrates and sugars), the keto diet adapts the body to a more sustainable source of energy that will fuel you for the long term rather than causing you to burn out quickly like a sugar high. Using keto intelligently leads to losing fat and dropping stubborn and unwanted pounds; the very fat you're trying to rid yourself of is used to fuel your weight loss. Research bears this out: Multiple studies show that people on carbohydrate-restricted diets, compared to low-fat and other "weight-loss diets," lose more weight in the first few months and successfully keep it off long term.

When you go into ketosis, you stop being a fat-making machine and instead become a fat-*burning* machine. Research shows that healthy young participants on a ketogenic diet increased their resting metabolism compared to others on a regular carbohydrate-indulgent diet. Interestingly, the more fat you have, the more you use; overweight people use a higher percentage of broken-down fatty acids as fuel than lean people. Going further, people on the standard ketogenic diet who eat up to 25 grams of daily carbs are able to lose weight, and more important, keep it off longer. This means that even a flexible keto diet will jump-start your weight loss.

The best part? The keto diet helps you lose weight while decreasing pesky cravings that are so common on low-fat diets. This way, you'll be more likely to go the distance in your weight loss journey. It may have to do with the fact that high-fat foods are just so satisfying that you'll naturally notice you're not as hungry as when you were eating more carbs or restricting your calories! The same is true of proteins, which are also a crucial part of the keto diet.

What's more, scientists are learning that ketones signal the body to eat less by affecting appetite hormones like ghrelin and leptin. These two hormones affect the body in opposite ways: Ghrelin levels typically rise when you're hungry to increase appetite, while leptin is turned on after a big meal, signaling your brain that it's time to stop eating. Research shows that ghrelin tends to rise when you cut calories to lose weight, which is why crash dieters find it so difficult to cut calories continuously. Ghrelin is screaming, "Eat!" and it's difficult to ignore. Ketosis, however, tends to block the increase in ghrelin, so you don't feel ravenous even when you're losing weight.

When you understand how ketosis works, this becomes intuitive. When the body feeds off of carbs, it quickly consumes them and then screams for more. When the body feeds off of fat, it utilizes all the consumed fat (what you just ate), and then when it's done, it naturally transitions to stored fat (what you were trying to get rid of in the first place). Your body stays satisfied because it's continuously feeding, and it's doing so off of the weight you want to lose!

This is vital to understand because many people who lose weight are not able to keep it off. In fact, most will end up packing on more pounds than they initially lost. This yo-yo dieting keeps many people in its grip, trying diet after diet, which only leads to feelings of deprivation, intense cravings, and inevitable overeating and rebound weight gain. That's not the case if you stick to a ketogenesis diet; your body doesn't stop burning fat over time, and your metabolism doesn't slow down as it would with low-fat diets.

REMEMBER

The keto diet is a natural and innovative way to jump-start your metabolism and turn you into a lean, fat-burning machine. Without the use of harmful chemicals or starvation diet techniques, you use your body's natural metabolic pathways to optimize your safe and long-term weight loss.

Improved body composition

Sculpting a lean body is one of the benefits that comes with keto weight loss. As we use our fat stores, we can whittle our waists, a vital sign of improved cardiovascular fitness. Belly fat is associated with heart disease, high blood pressure, and diabetes. It's no secret that, as we age, many of us tend to lose muscle and gain fat. Ketosis stops this in its tracks. By using fat as fuel and providing adequate protein, people on the keto diet maintain their lean muscle mass over the long term because it's not used as a source of energy.

A few studies have looked at the changes in body fat and lean muscle mass when the ketogenic diet is combined with exercise. In two studies, participants on the keto diet (70 percent to 75 percent of calories from fat, 20 percent from protein, and less than 10 percent from carbohydrates) lost more total body fat and belly fat than men on the same strength-based routines who ate a typical carbohydrate-rich diet (50 percent to 55 percent calories from carbohydrates, 25 percent from fat, and 20 percent from protein). The results regarding lean muscle mass were mixed; in the longer study, the keto diet nearly doubled lean body mass, while in the other study, there was no change in this area.

When accompanied by increased resistance training, only the ketogenic diet led to total body fat loss. This is incredibly important for athletes, who may want to decrease body fat percentage — an essential concept in many athletic sports — rather than just lose weight. As such, the ketogenic diet is a safer option for meeting weigh-in requirements or obtaining a "sculpted" shape for competitive sports such as bodybuilding. Importantly, it does not do this at the cost of restricting much-needed calories, as may happen in athletes desperate to lose weight quickly. Therefore, there is little risk of muscle loss and fatigue and a high chance of weight loss.

These studies showed that the ketogenic diet is unlikely to cause an absolute increase in muscle mass. *Lean body mass* (the body weight that is not made up of fat) may increase, or at worst stay the same with the ketogenic diet, but you're unlikely to bulk up. One of the critical factors in building muscle mass is maintaining an excess of protein in your system so your body can use it as building blocks. When you consume too much protein, your body can use a process called *gluconeogenesis* to convert some of the protein to glucose, knocking you out of keto.

REMEMBER

Unlike unhealthy performance enhancers or diet drugs, the keto diet effectively helps you lose body fat while maintaining your hard-earned muscle. It's safe to use for both extreme athletes and weekend warriors because it gives you adequate protein to protect you from muscle loss while providing fat to fuel your metabolism through sustained exercise.

Increased energy

A common misperception is that ketosis tricks your body into thinking it's starving. Although ketosis shares some traits with starvation, your body is not starving, and you aren't hypoglycemic. This means you won't have dangerous lows in your sugar levels that can leave you feeling lethargic, weak, and "hangry." Many people, especially well-meaning physicians or nutritionists who aren't familiar with the diet, worry that ketosis will lead to a permanent state of exhaustion and lethargy. This just isn't true — your blood glucose levels will naturally be in the low end of the normal range because your body isn't using glucose as its primary fuel; it's using ketones. This is the ideal way to reduce your risk for diabetes and cardiovascular disease, which are common factors that cause your body to feel exhausted all the time.

Compared to other options, the keto diet is more likely to improve your energy and sense of vitality. In a study looking at older individuals with type 2 diabetes who followed a keto diet over two years, researchers noticed an overall improvement in their quality of life compared to those who stuck to the low-fat diet. Specifically, those in the keto group:

>> Were better equipped to complete daily activities and chores

>> Experienced increased energy levels

>> Minimized routine body aches and pains

In addition to providing an excellent source of energy, the keto diet may just bump up your mood. Ketones affect the levels of neurotransmitters important for mood regulation, such as gamma-aminobutyric acid (GABA) and monoamines. A growing body of evidence suggests that a keto diet may help decrease depression and relieve anxiety. Overall, compared to a low-fat diet, multiple studies prove that people feel better on a keto diet.

Concerned that you won't be able to keep up with your usual activities or start training for a hike or a marathon? Whether you're trying to build up your endurance or you're an Olympic athlete, the keto diet won't affect your stamina and may even increase it. A study from the 1980s that examined overweight individuals found that, after adapting to the ketogenic diet over six weeks, participants were able to increase the intensity of a treadmill workout while decreasing the amount of effort they used to accomplish it.

The same goes for athletes: Those who enter ketosis (for example, practicing Muslims who fast during the month of Ramadan) had no adverse effects on their level of physical fitness, nor did they complain about lower energy levels during training (after the requisite period of adjustment to ketosis). In the same vein, studies of high-level athletes who ate an adequate amount of protein for their exercise levels on the ketogenic diet showed that they were able to maintain stable levels of endurance and strength performance without the need to refuel on high-carb snacks.

REMEMBER

Fat fuels your body. On the keto diet, your glucose levels remain in a healthy range so you aren't risking the dangerous rollercoaster blood sugar levels that can leave you lethargic, irritable, and just plain unhappy. Keto gets it right by keeping both your brain and your muscles efficient and energetic.

Improved mental focus

Ketosis is a natural way to achieve a clear and focused mental state, an achievement your brain will thank you for. Ketones are an efficient nutrition source for your body, feeding into the energy-making pathway (known as the *Krebs cycle*) more quickly than glucose, which must take a circuitous path to produce energy. Using such an intelligent system naturally has a positive effect on the brain. Ketones stimulate *neurotrophins,* proteins that increase growth and development of brain cells or neurons. They improve neurons' resistance to the stress of daily life and are involved in promoting our synaptic connections, which are vital for memory and learning.

Although using the ketogenic diet to treat conditions other than epilepsy is still a blossoming field, studies in mice show that ketosis improves their ability to learn and make new memories. A few studies in humans show that people on a ketogenic diet are able to process information faster. Ketones effectively target the brain's hippocampus, which is a critical part of the ability to learn new facts as well as remember them later. This suggests that a keto lifestyle could leave you better able to deal with the million tasks at hand at any given moment.

There is a lot of excitement that the keto diet may help treat neurodegenerative diseases, the all-too-common disorders associated with premature aging and malfunction of the brain and spinal cord. Because ketosis is such an efficient cellular process, scientists think it may be a helpful tool to prevent and perhaps eventually cure neurodegenerative conditions, which are often caused by metabolic inefficiency in the brain. Ketones increase adenosine triphosphate (ATP), the body's energy currency, and decrease signs of inflammation in brain tissue. Keto diets are being offered to people with Alzheimer's, and the results are remarkable.

Alzheimer's is the most common neurodegenerative disease and the leading cause of dementia in the elderly. Despite a progressive decline in function in the face of current medications, research shows that inducing ketosis in rat models is able to remove abnormal proteins characteristically found in the brains of people with Alzheimer's. Medium-chain triglyceride (MCT) supplements improved Alzheimer's patients' ability to recall a paragraph they had just read, which is an important milestone. Similar benefits are being discovered in other neurodegenerative disorders like Parkinson's disease and even traumatic brain injury.

REMEMBER

Ketones are an excellent source of fuel for your brain. A ketogenic diet can lead you to work smarter, rather than harder, and may be a key target for improving and even reversing neurodegenerative diseases.

Better sleep

Sleep is an incredibly crucial determining factor in our ability to stay energetic and mentally focused throughout the day. Anyone who has struggled with insomnia understands the incredible importance of sleep. It allows us to incorporate new information into our brains and store it in our long-term memory. In short, without rest, we can't learn new things. The body cycles through four different stages of sleep several times a night:

>> **Stage 1:** The lightest of the sleep stages. Most people can be woken easily from this level of unconsciousness by a loud sound or other kind of interruption.

>> **Stage 2:** In this stage, your body begins to transition to the deeper cycles. Your heart rate slows, body temperature decreases, and breathing gets deeper.

>> **Stage 3:** The most restorative stage of sleep. It's very difficult to awaken someone in this state.

>> **Rapid eye movement (REM) sleep:** Also known as dreaming, this stage of sleep helps to incorporate skills and controls the emotional aspects of memory.

You need all types of sleep to function properly. When you miss vital parts of sleep, you're left not only exhausted and fatigued but also unable to make decisions and think straight, and you're even depressed and can face a general sense of impotence in life.

Ketosis may not only help you get to sleep, but it can likely improve the quality of your sleep while decreasing the overall amount you need. How's that for efficiency? Most of the studies looking at this issue studied people with seizures or other neurological problems, but the findings are likely applicable to the rest of us. In one of these studies, the keto diet not only decreased the amount of time children with epilepsy slept, but also simultaneously increased the total amount of REM sleep while maintaining the amount of deep sleep. This means more time was spent in the crucial areas of sleep rather than the light stages of sleep, which are not as restful and are also the stages in which you're more likely to wake up accidentally. A year later, these same participants needed fewer naps, experienced fewer seizures, and maintained the increased time in REM sleep.

Although the specific mechanism of how ketones affect sleep is not known, the fact remains that you can improve the effectiveness of your sleep by changing the way you eat.

Stabilized blood sugar

Ketosis is, by definition, a state of perfect glucose control. Carbs and processed sugars cause diabetes and glucose intolerance, the precursor to diabetes. About one-third of Americans are prediabetic but don't know it, and these Americans are unlikely to be on the ketogenic diet.

Complex carbs (like potatoes, bread, and rice), although they seem healthier than refined sugar, are still turned into glucose by your body and increase your insulin resistance. By decreasing overall carbs as the keto diet recommends, you bypass this unhealthy cycle of constantly shuttling glucose in and out of your cells. On the ketogenic diet, your glucose levels are neither too high nor too low but maintained in a perfect and low normal range.

Doctors know that these wide swings in sugar levels, even if your body initially manages them well, will lead to inflammation and decreased insulin sensitivity over time. The constant up and down of insulin secretion affects the pancreas, leaving it drained and unable to keep up with the load of carbs it continually sees. High levels of insulin can cause real harm; excess insulin is often a precursor to diabetes and sign of insulin insensitivity, which is associated with inflammation and obesity even in people without diabetes.

Recent research shows that people with type 2 diabetes do much better on a low-carb diet than the low-fat diet many doctors have recommended in the past. In fact, multiple studies show that diabetic people who are on the ketogenic diet significantly lower their blood sugar levels to the point that they can drastically decrease or even get rid of the medications that they thought would be lifelong. This is because eating a truly ketogenic diet is the same as not eating insulin-provoking carbs — there is almost no appreciable change in blood sugar levels or insulin levels.

Compare that to eating even the "healthiest" of carbohydrates, and you'll notice a drastic difference in the sugar levels. "Healthy carbs" are those with a low glycemic index, a food rating system that evaluates the effect of a food on blood sugar levels. Low-glycemic-index foods are considered healthy, but low-carb, low-glycemic-index foods are even better.

Healthier cholesterol levels

Cholesterol often gets a bad name in nutrition circles, but it's a necessary part of the human body. Cholesterol is a component of cell membranes and steroid hormones, and it's even vital for moving cholesterol out of our blood vessels where it can cause damage and lead to atherosclerosis or heart disease. There are several categories of cholesterol:

>> **Total cholesterol:** The total amount of cholesterol in your blood. This number on a lab report adds up the following two categories and presents them as a single number:

  - **Low-density lipoprotein (LDL):** Often referred to as "bad" cholesterol. LDL is commonly associated with conditions like diabetes, strokes, and heart attacks.

  - **High-density lipoprotein (HDL):** Often referred to as "good" cholesterol. High levels of HDL are just the opposite of LDL; they tend to protect against diabetes, strokes, and heart attacks.

>> **Triglycerides:** Fats that are freely floating in your blood. These levels should rise when you eat a fatty meal but should go down to normal when you're fasting.

Although all these blood tests are associated with fats, the truth is that improving blood sugar control — by decreasing carb intake — is the most critical thing you can do to improve these numbers. By following a low-carb diet, you can lower your total cholesterol levels (primarily made up of LDL) and triglycerides, while raising HDL. It also improves the ratio of HDL to total cholesterol, another important marker of heart health.

Another way the keto diet keeps you healthy is by blocking the cholesterol-producing enzyme called *HMG-CoA reductase,* an enzyme that stimulates the liver to make more cholesterol, beyond the cholesterol you eat. Reducing your carb intake naturally blocks the enzyme's function. This enzyme is the same one that is blocked by the common medicines, statins — the most commonly prescribed medication to improve cholesterol levels. Statins are so prevalent, in fact, that some doctors think everyone should be on a statin. In reality, everyone can naturally reduce his or her cholesterol by eating a healthy keto diet, without the many side effects associated with taking a statin.

REMEMBER

Socrates was on to something when he said, "Let food be thy medicine." By eating a healthy keto diet, you're doing just that: improving your cholesterol levels with real food, not engineered pharmaceuticals.

Reduced blood pressure

The ketogenic diet is often mistakenly thought of as a high protein diet, but it isn't. The typical diet is a moderate protein diet that allows protein in the amount of 0.36 gram of protein per pound of body weight, which is what the moderately active person would typically need. A benefit of the keto diet is that the *amino acids* (protein building blocks) that are involved in ketosis are often blood-pressure-lowering proteins as opposed to acidifying amino acids, which are found in other metabolic states.

Keto is often oversimplified as a bacon and cheese diet, which relies heavily on salt-rich foods that may increase the risk of high blood pressure in susceptible people. Generally speaking, Americans eat too much salt; we need only about 500 milligrams per day, and the average American gets more than 3,000 milligrams (to put that in perspective, 1 teaspoon of salt is equal to 2,300 milligrams). That excess salt is associated with long-term high blood pressure in people who have family members with high blood pressure or other risk factors. Interestingly, ketosis actually can lead to decreases in the amount of salt your body retains. Many processed-carb foods are actually high in salt and are effectively cut out in the ketogenic diet. In fact, many people on keto can actually indulge in adding salt because they're much more likely to be closer to or lower than the recommended salt levels than the average American.

Reduced acne

Ever notice how a night out on the town with one too many cocktails, or perhaps a candy binge over Halloween shows up the next day on your skin? You're not alone — acne commonly happens to people eating a high-sugar diet. On the other hand, acne is almost rare in non-Westerners who don't eat a high-sugar diet. When you change the low-sugar group's diet and switch them to eating sugar-sweetened breakfast cereals and granola bars, the acne pops up. Studies show that people with acne tend to eat more carbs with high-glycemic-index foods and have higher levels of insulin and insulin-like growth factor.

High-glycemic-index foods, the ones that dramatically raise your blood sugar and insulin levels, not only increase your risk of glucose intolerance and diabetes, but also affect your skin. High insulin sets up a cascade of effects, which can lead to increased inflammation in skin cells. Interestingly, women who have polycystic ovarian syndrome (PCOS) — a type of insulin insensitivity — are more likely than their peers to have acne.

Dermatologists and their patients with acne scars are catching on to this link and are seeing a benefit after switching to a low-carb eating style. Multiple studies of people with moderate or severe acne showed that sticking to a keto-like diet is associated with a decrease in severity of acne and acne scars, even when you don't buy expensive skin products or wash your face five times a day.

Acne is a physical manifestation of the inflammation that is going on in your body. Many dermatologists and beauty insiders believe that the skin provides insight into the overall health of your body. Flares of acne and skin irritation suggest that your body is struggling with health, and they can be your body telling you something is wrong.

TIP

Acne may be more than skin deep. If you're having breakout after breakout and nothing, not even top-grade beauty products, is working, it may be time to look deeper at why your skin is so inflamed. It may just be all those excess carbohydrates.

Less inflammation

As mentioned earlier, the keto diet is not new. Although it was popularized in the 1920s for specific medical conditions, it has been a way of life for generations in some cultures. The fact is that ketones, especially β-hydroxybutyrate, the main ketone in your body, are anti-inflammatory. Inflammation, specifically low-grade chronic inflammation, seems to be the basis for many of the so-called disease of our modern age. Studies show that infusing mice with these magic ketones decreases a variety of inflammation-associated illnesses, ranging from Alzheimer's to type 2 diabetes and atherosclerosis.

In fact, keto simulates our evolutionary beginnings, when food was not so readily available. The keto diet shares some similarities to starvation (even though you aren't starving) and forces the body to use alternate pathways and processes that allow it to thrive. Some evolutionary biologists suggest that the keto diet is a culmination of evolution's attempt to increases our longevity and fight disease. Unfortunately, as we've drastically changed our diet and moved away from keto over the last hundred or so years, our biology has responded with inflammation-based illnesses that are pleading with us to change our ways.

Health benefits

One of the most fascinating aspects of keto is how it works *with* the body to create better health and combat a number of known diseases and conditions. Many of these health issues are either directly created or exacerbated by excess carbohydrates, so switching from a glucose-based diet to a ketones-based diet addresses multiple health issues without intentionally targeting them.

Epilepsy

Although not commonly known, the keto diet was first used in the United States to treat epilepsy. Doctors in the 1920s realized that children with intractable epilepsy showed drastic improvement when they fasted.

Obviously, starvation is not a good idea long term, but doctors discovered that a high-fat, low-carb diet, like starvation, led to ketosis. By placing children on this diet, their seizures — which were so severe that they became mentally incapacitated — resolved. Johns Hopkins has an integrative clinic that uses a very strict keto diet to treat patients who have no other options. The diet is still used for these children and is now approved for rare forms of seizures that have no cure and don't respond to traditional anti-seizure medications.

Diabetes and other metabolic disorders

Diabetes is a growing epidemic in our society. One in ten people around the world have the disease, and it's often associated with other metabolic issues such as high blood pressure, abnormal cholesterol levels, and insulin resistance, collectively known as *metabolic syndrome.* The keto diet can treat and even reverse type 2 diabetes and metabolic syndrome. High intake of carbohydrates and glucose leads to insulin insufficiency, or prediabetes, a condition which now affects about one-third of Americans. People with prediabetes are more likely to turn glucose into fat, which leads to worsening of their overall health.

However, when people with diabetes switch to a low-carb diet like keto, they lower their blood glucose levels and improve the standard blood marker for diabetes, hemoglobin A1c (HgbA1c). In fact, diabetics who stick to the keto diet are often able to reverse their diabetes and stop taking medications. Doctors figured this out as long ago as the 1970s, yet many people with diabetes are still not aware of the significant steps they can choose to take control of their health. This holds true regardless of how much weight a person with diabetes loses, which is a common recommendation for improving blood sugar levels.

An important caveat is that while the keto diet may have significant benefits for type 2 diabetes, it is not explicitly recommended for people within type 1 diabetes, the form of diabetes often seen in children and teens. Compared to type 2 diabetes, which causes insulin insensitivity, people with type 1 diabetes don't make insulin at all.

Fibromyalgia

Fibromyalgia is a chronic pain condition that affects millions of people worldwide. Unfortunately, it's also a "catch-all" term used when doctors and other medical professionals aren't sure how to treat chronic pain, leading many people to suffer. Pain medications and incomplete remedies only partially mask the problem.

Many researchers believe that an underlying cause of fibromyalgia is constant inflammation, which depends on the food that enters our mouths. Many people with fibromyalgia have sugar and hormone imbalances, over-excited pain sensors, free radicals, and poor liver function. All these conditions wreak havoc on the body, causing neurons to fire repeatedly, eventually leading to damage. Poor liver health, which blocks your body's ability to get rid of toxins or inflammatory particles (like free radicals), further damages our pain nerves and muscles, causing us to feel pain with no trigger.

When you change your diet by removing harmful high-carb and high-sugar foods that turn into fat, you reverse hormonal imbalances and attack the inflammatory cause of fibromyalgia pain. Studies show that an increase in carbohydrate intake often leads to worse outcomes in people with fibromyalgia. This is separate from the associated pain with being overweight.

Many people with fibromyalgia are overweight and experience increasing pain from arthritis, another inflammatory condition. As you can imagine, all this inflammation only worsens pain. Not only can the ketogenic diet help with weight loss, but it also gets rid of many of the problems caused by too much sugar. In a study using animal models, scientists discovered that a ketogenic diet actually reduced symptoms of chronic pain. They found that ketone metabolism is less inflammatory than a carbohydrate-based diet and decreases the activity of pain fiber, which is one of the things that tricks us into thinking we're in pain. What's more, it appears that the underlying benefit is similar to keto's success with epilepsy. Keto increases both adenosine and gamma-aminobutyric acid (GABA), two powerful inhibitory substances in the nervous system that help to decrease our response to and sensation of pain.

Cardiovascular disease

Keto, and fat overall, are great for your heart. The keto diet

>> Helps you maintain a healthy weight

>> Improves blood sugar control

>> Improves your blood cholesterol levels

>> Is anti-inflammatory

All these actions help to decrease the two most common results of heart disease: heart attacks and strokes. Research supports this: Studies show that people eating a healthy, whole-foods, low-carb diet have a decreased risk of cardiovascular disease.

Potential Drawbacks of the Keto Diet

Unfortunately, there are some growing pains associated with switching to a keto diet. But as we know, nothing that is worth it is easy (although it does get easier). Your body is used to its steady supply of carbohydrates and glucose, and there will be a bit of a transition period until the body adjusts to its new source of fuel. Knowing what to expect makes things easier, so here are a few things to be aware of on your journey to keto lifestyle.

Keto flu

The *keto flu* is a well-known deterrent for some people beginning the keto journey. Some, but not all, people who begin a very low-carbohydrate lifestyle complain about feeling like they have the flu during the first several days of starting the keto diet. Signs of keto flu are

>> Brain fog

>> Constipation

>> Feeling tired all the time

>> Muscle aches and pain

>> Poor sleep quality

Many people notice the first few days or weeks of switching to a keto diet can be rough. As you drastically cut back on sugars and switch to fat as your primary energy source, your body must become accustomed to a world with lower glucose levels. This causes a decrease in body water as your carbohydrate stores (which retain water) are lost. As you lose body water, you also lose salt, which can worsen the feeling of fatigue and weakness. Potassium levels can drop as well. You may feel the low potassium levels as muscle aches, which are common symptoms of the flu.

Additionally, sugar is essentially an addictive drug. Studies show that sugar activates the body's endocannabinoid system — the same system that strong painkillers and heroin use. It's no wonder that a sudden loss of the sugar "drug" causes you to have intense cravings.

TIP

There are a few tricks to get through the keto flu:

>> **Keep up with your potassium and magnesium intake.** You can load up on avocados (good sources of both), but it's a good idea to take a multivitamin around this time to make sure you're meeting your daily requirement. Both minerals also help to reduce muscle cramping associated with keto flu.

- » **Replenish lost salt.** Drink broth, use your salt shaker, and even add salt to your water.

- » **Stay hydrated.** This is crucial to getting over the dehydration of keto flu.

- » **Get rest.** Your body is going through a lot of changes; rest will help with recovery. Good sleep also helps to reduce levels of *cortisol* (the fight-or-flight hormone that is associated with inflammation) in your body.

- » **Take a break from strenuous exercise.** Exercise is an integral part of healthy living, but now is not the time to run a marathon or go sign up for CrossFit. You can generally maintain your current activity levels, although your performance may drop for a couple of weeks.

- » **Take a fiber supplement.** There are many low-carb, high-fiber foods, but you may need a supplement in the early days of transition.

Over time, as your body gets used to ketosis, the keto flu will resolve. Generally, it lasts between four days and a week. The rebound is increased energy and even improved mood.

Keto breath

Some people notice a sweet, "fruity" breath after being on the keto diet. In some people, the odor is more like nail polish remover. This is nothing to be alarmed about, and it will eventually resolve itself. *Keto breath* is caused by acetone, one of the three ketones of ketosis.

Acetone does not have any significant health benefits compared to the other two common ketones of ketosis (β-hydroxybutyric acid and acetoacetate), but its characteristic odor is a useful marker for ketosis. Keto breath is also common in ketosis from starvation, strenuous exercise, and even *ketoacidosis*, a metabolic state when your body pushes past ketosis and becomes unhealthy.

Ketoacidosis

Although the names are similar, ketosis is not the same as ketoacidosis. Ketoacidosis is essentially ketosis gone awry and is most commonly encountered by people who have a problem with insulin deficiency, like type 1 diabetics. Ketoacidosis often occurs in people with severe diabetes, when their insulin just can't keep up with the amount of sugar in the bloodstream. The body turns to fat as a source of fuel, but the difference is that it does this in the presence of a lot of sugar, and to a level that is toxic to the body. People who are in ketoacidosis have blood ketone levels of more than 25 mmol, whereas people in ketosis have levels that are less than 7 or 8 mmol. (People on a standard, carb-heavy diet have a level about 0.1 mmol.)

The difference in the amount of ketosis makes a huge difference. The high and abnormal levels of ketones cause *acidosis,* which means the blood is too acidic, affecting its ability to function normally. Ketoacidosis leads to severe dehydration, confusion, vomiting, and belly pain. People with ketoacidosis may lose consciousness and need to be hospitalized. This is different from the keto diet, because in ketosis, you efficiently use your ketones for energy, not allowing the levels to rise to the point that is harmful to your body. People in ketoacidosis develop symptoms quickly and get sick very quickly. It's extremely rare for a healthy person without prediabetes or diabetes to go into ketoacidosis.

REMEMBER

Ketoacidosis is ketosis gone wrong; it happens most often in people who are on high-carb diets and whose bodies can't process very high levels of blood sugar, causing them to turn to ketones in desperation. A person on the keto diet who doesn't have these preexisting conditions should never encounter ketoacidosis.

Nutritional deficiencies

Switching to a ketogenic diet requires you to drastically shift the variety of foods you eat and (initially) you may lose out on some nutrients found in carbohydrate-rich foods. For example, people on a ketogenic diet tend to lose potassium naturally and may be unaware of keto-friendly potassium sources like cooked leafy greens and avocados. As you learn to eat a range of healthy keto foods, it's essential to have a buffer to get you through the change. A multivitamin is helpful in this regard — assuming you choose one without added sugars (a common additive in vitamins and supplements).

As you become more acquainted with the keto lifestyle and incorporate vitamin-rich, low-carb veggies and a range of healthy whole foods, the need for a multivitamin may go away. Two other beneficial supplements for the keto lifestyle are fiber and MCT oil. Again, fiber often comes packaged with starchy carbohydrates, which are off-limits to keto folks. Taking a fiber supplement or a tablespoon of MCT oil can help address things like constipation early on. We cover the best supplements in Chapter 8.

The Lowdown on Fat and Cholesterol

Both fat and cholesterol suffer from more than their fair share of myths, misinformation, and misconceptions. Fat is a critical macronutrient, and the body can't survive without it, despite the impressions you may have from the food and diet campaigns of the 1990s. Cholesterol is also crucial to maintaining a healthy body, although there are several types of cholesterol and knowing the difference (and how you can affect the numbers) is very important.

Identifying the real villains: Sugar and processed foods

If you read this far, you likely know where this is heading: Eating a ketogenic diet — high in fat and low in carbohydrates — will not make you fat. Instead, it will probably help you *shed* unwanted pounds. This myth that "fat makes you fat" only rings true when the high-fat foods come with a high amount of carbohydrates.

Instead, the underlying culprit for fat gain is carbohydrates. This is becoming more apparent as we realize that the popularity of the low-fat diet of the 1990s coincided with an astronomical increase in rates of obesity and diabetes. Drinking a can of soda a day — a low-fat, high-carb option — increases your risk of diabetes. Carbs are addicting fuel: Sugar triggers the brain in the same way as opiates do, making you want more and more. As too many of us know, this can quickly spiral out of control, leading to carb binges that leave you feeling bloated, depleted, and awful.

TIP

The real villain making you fat is the excess carbs you're eating. Decreasing carbs rather than fat will get you closer to your weight-loss goals.

Taking the blame off dietary fat

Fat is an essential macronutrient, unlike carbohydrates. You need fat to survive, whereas your body (through a process called *gluconeogenesis*; see Chapter 3) can make all the carbohydrates your body needs. Fat, including cholesterol, is vital for a well-functioning body. It allows brain signals to move smoothly, is a critical component of cell membranes, and is crucial for a host of hormones the body needs to communicate internally. Without fat, we become a shell of our highly functioning selves. It's only recently, within the past several decades, that we have removed fat from our food and replaced it with sugars, leading to a host of illnesses such as chronic inflammation, diabetes, obesity, and more.

On the keto diet, you learn about all the benefits a wide array of healthy fats provides. Over time, you'll relish using olive oil as the basis of your salad dressing, rather than low-fat ranch, or treating yourself with an avocado-based pudding, rather than the sugar-infused Jell-O. The possibilities with fats are endless!

Exposing the truth about cholesterol

There is quite a bit of controversy about cholesterol. Cholesterol is an integral part of the human body, yet most people think they need to stay far away from it. The fact is, a keto diet helps to improve cholesterol levels. When you eat cholesterol-rich food, you're primed to think that it will raise "bad" cholesterol (LDL), but that just isn't the case. Eating cholesterol doesn't immediately translate to having a bad score on your cholesterol test. More and more studies show that high-carb diets are more likely to raise your cholesterol than eating dietary cholesterol.

What's more, LDL is a little more complicated than most doctors initially thought. Although it's called "bad" cholesterol, it isn't that simple. LDL is a combination of many different types of cholesterol, and scientists have found that only some types of LDL — not the whole group — are bad for the heart. Although the ketogenic diet can raise overall LDL levels, it tends only to raise the "good" kind, called LDL-C. LDL-C are "fluffy" molecules that are less likely to clog your arteries and, therefore, less likely to lead to *atherosclerosis* (hardening of the arteries) than the smaller and denser LDL, which are bad for you. So, although on the surface the keto diet may raise your LDL levels, it does it in the healthiest way possible. On the other hand, most carbohydrates increase the small, dense LDL, while decreasing heart-friendly HDL.

Of course, as we mention earlier it's a good idea to get a wide range of fats in a keto diet because some healthy fats, like olive oil, are great at raising heart-healthy HDL.

REMEMBER

Dietary cholesterol is not your enemy. If something is raising your cholesterol levels, it's more likely that the blame rests with high-carb and processed foods.

Chapter **3**

Understanding What Happens to Your Body in Ketosis

To succeed on the keto diet, you need to understand how your body uses and stores energy from food. The human body is amazingly intelligent and adaptable, using available resources to create the energy it needs to survive in whatever environment it encounters.

Over hundreds of thousands of years of evolution, humans have devised intricate and finely tuned processes to turn the food we put into our bodies into energy that allows us to play musical instruments, run marathons, or sit quietly and contemplate life. We derive this energy from *macronutrients* (commonly called *macros*), the basic components of food that provide energy in the form of calories. The macronutrients are carbohydrates, fats, and proteins.

In this chapter, we fill you in on how your body uses macros for fuel, as well as the changes that happen when you're eating normally, fasting, or starving. We also touch on what to expect after switching to the keto lifestyle, both at the beginning and down the road, and we fill you in on how to figure out if you're in ketosis.

Exploring Your Body's Flex-Fuel System

If you've spent some time underneath the hood of your car, you've probably heard of flex-fuel systems: engines that can pick and choose which fuel to run on. Similarly, the human body is flexible when it comes to the type of fuel it uses. Your body can run on fat or carbohydrates, and you get to make a choice with each bite you take. In this section, we walk you through the different fuels the body uses and how it affects how well you "run."

Burning carbs: Glycolysis

Without a doubt, carbohydrates are the most consumed macronutrients around the world, encompassing upwards of 50 percent of all calories for most humans. However, it hasn't always been this way. How humans eat has shifted drastically over the last hundred years as food has increasingly become industrially produced and refined, allowing the lowly carbohydrate to become the most consumed macronutrient around the world.

Regardless, carbohydrates are used in the body to produce energy at a rate of 4 calories per gram. All carbs are eventually turned into glucose, the smallest unit of carbohydrates. No matter what type of carbohydrate you eat, whether it's a cup of whole grain oats or a cube of sugar, your blood sugar will rise as the starch is broken down into glucose and enters the bloodstream.

The process of turning glucose into energy begins with *glycolysis*, the first step in the complex sequence of events that transforms glucose into energy the body can use. Insulin levels rise when increased glycolysis is happening, and is the hormone that stops functioning or is lost in people with diabetes. Insulin is needed for cells to take up glucose for energy; without insulin, cells are like a fish out of water, surrounded by the very thing they need (energy) but with no way to use it. When too much insulin is present, your system gets used to it and requires more and more for the same effect — this is called *insulin resistance.* One of the major benefits of keto is that your system gets a break from insulin; over time, that insulin sensitivity returns, restoring the person's health.

After insulin does its job, glucose enters the cells and can get to work providing fuel for your body. Virtually every cell in your body can use glucose for energy. Even your fat cells need glucose to store fat! One of insulin's roles is to act as a signal to tell your body to increase its fat stores.

You don't have to eat carbohydrates from food for your body to find the glucose it needs. Your body is capable of generating all the glucose it needs through a process called *gluconeogenesis,* which primarily happens in the liver, and to some smaller degree, the kidneys. These organs then export the glucose to the other parts of the body that need it for energy.

REMEMBER

Your body treats all carbohydrates, whether they're "good" carbs or "bad" carbs, the same way. Carbohydrates cause a spike in insulin that ultimately increases your risk for diabetes and encourages your body to pack on the pounds.

Burning fat: Ketosis

Ketosis is the process your body uses to breaks down ketone bodies for most of its energy needs. Ketones come from fatty acids regardless of whether you eat them or get them from your fat cells. Your body prefers to use glucose for energy (see the preceding section), so ketosis only occurs when you don't have enough glucose coming in from your diet. On a keto diet, your body switches from glycolysis to ketosis as the primary energy generator.

Fat, like carbohydrates, is also a source of calories, but it provides a whopping nine calories per gram, compared to the measly four calories you get from carbs and protein. This means, head to head, fat is always a more efficient source of energy than carbohydrates.

On the keto diet, instead of using glycolysis for energy, fatty acids are broken down into three types of ketones that provide energy to all your body's cells:

>> **Acetoacetate:** The main ketone made by your liver.

>> **β-hydroxybutyric acid:** The main ketone in your bloodstream and the source of ketones' anti-inflammatory benefits.

>> **Acetone:** The least common ketone; it doesn't provide energy, but it is responsible for carrying waste out of the body. It's responsible for *keto breath* (the fruity or moldy breath that some people have when in ketosis) because it's ridding the body of excess acetone through the lungs.

Importantly, fatty acids not only make ketones but also are able to produce glucose if you aren't getting it from your diet. That's why, even on the keto diet, your blood sugar levels don't drop precipitously. They also don't rise astronomically, as they do on a carb-rich diet, every time you take a bite of food.

The liver, the workhorse of metabolism, can't use ketones as its energy source, so it's crucial that fat can be turned into glucose to support the liver during ketosis. Like glucose, ketones are also a source of energy for the brain and provide its fuel during ketosis. Ketones may be better brain fuel than carbohydrates because they've been shown to improve the health of our brain cells and may be helpful in preventing neurodegenerative diseases like Alzheimer's.

TECHNICAL STUFF

The words *ketosis, ketogenesis,* and *ketogenic* are all derived from a similar root, meaning to produce and utilize ketone bodies as the primary form of energy. That's where the names *ketogenic diet* and *keto diet* come from!

Burning protein: Gluconeogenesis

Protein is the least preferred source of energy. Your body prefers to use proteins to build tissues and organs, as well as regulate many of the normal functions of the body. Insulin, the hormone that regulates glucose, is a protein. Protein is the last resource for producing energy because breaking it down means taking protein from your muscles and slowing down the key processes your body relies on to function properly.

Regardless, proteins do provide energy at the same level as carbohydrates, which is four calories per gram. Protein becomes an energy source when you:

>> Starve.

>> Eat a very high-protein diet.

>> Switch from a high-carbohydrate lifestyle to a keto lifestyle.

Amino acids (the building block of proteins) can be converted into glucose, through a process called *gluconeogenesis.* Proteins are not the only starting point for gluconeogenesis — fats and other substances can also be used to make glucose. However, gluconeogenesis, especially with protein as its source, requires energy, making protein an expensive and ineffective source of fuel.

REMEMBER

Most proteins cause a (moderate) spike in insulin levels. The spike is not nearly as high as the one you get from eating carbohydrates, but it's still there. That's why the keto diet is a "moderate protein" diet. Adding excess proteins (more than your body needs) to your diet decreases the benefits of the very-low-carbohydrate lifestyle by adding insulin back into the equation.

Following the Energy Flow along the Metabolic Pathways

In this section, we walk you through energy production in the human body, both when you're on a standard high-carbohydrate diet and when you're on a very low-carbohydrate keto diet. This section helps you understand the importance of the sources of your calories and exposes the fallacy of the idea that "a calorie is a calorie." Where you get your calories from, not just how many of them you consume, is essential.

When food is available

Let's look at what happens when you eat a meal. You're eating, so fuel is easy to come by, and your body makes the most of the readily available calories.

Standard high-carbohydrate diet

When you eat a carbohydrate-rich meal, your saliva and intestines have to break down the carbohydrates into glucose (through many enzymes) so that it can be absorbed and used for fuel. This is why carbohydrates, whether they're simple (like a soda) or complex (like whole-grain oatmeal), are treated similarly by the body: They all turn into glucose, no matter what they look like on your plate.

As glucose enters the body, it signals the pancreas to make *insulin*, the hormone that moves glucose into your body's cells. High glucose levels are harmful, causing a buildup of acid and unhealthy fluid shifts in the blood. Insulin rushes into the bloodstream to lower glucose levels and keep your blood healthy.

Releasing insulin is a necessary reaction to glucose in your blood, but over time this becomes problematic. If you eat sugar over and over, your body may have a hard time figuring out exactly how much insulin to release. Swings in insulin lead to significant changes in blood sugar over time, which can leave you feeling "hangry" (when sugar levels are low) at one moment and lethargic (when sugar levels are high) at the next.

Over time, your body develops a tolerance for insulin, and you need more of it to have the same effect. This is the beginning of insulin insensitivity or insulin resistance and is a definite step on the pathway toward type 2 diabetes. Insulin not only brings glucose into your cells but also instructs your fat cells to grow: Your body assumes that there is a lot of readily available energy and is intelligently trying to save your fat for the possible lean times ahead. When it's inside the cell, glucose provides energy to your cells or is stored for future use (in the liver and muscle).

Your body can't store much glucose — only about a day's worth of calories is stored as *glycogen* (the storage form of glucose). Your body, however, can quickly turn excess glucose into fat, which can be stored in limitless supply, as anyone struggling with weight loss knows all too well.

Keto diet

When you follow a keto diet, there aren't many carbohydrates around, so glucose levels don't increase in your blood. Instead, the fats you eat are broken down into triglycerides and *fatty acids,* the fundamental component of fat. These components are then carried to the liver and broken down into ketone bodies, which are then used to produce energy in your body's cells. Almost every organ in your body (exceptions include the liver and red blood cells) can use ketones for the energy it needs.

The difference between high-carb and keto diets is that there is no spike in blood glucose levels with the latter. During ketosis, high glucose levels can't potentially damage the body and insulin levels don't rise, so you're not primed to store fat. In fact, the opposite happens: Low levels of glucose and insulin encourage your body to break down fat from your food and your fat cells to serve as the source of energy your body needs.

REMEMBER

The ketogenic diet combines the benefits of low carbohydrates and low insulin with the energy benefits of using ketones as the primary source of fuel. It's a win-win situation.

When the body is in fasting mode

Next, what happens after you've eaten and absorbed your meal, and your body has to rely on its reserves? You may be surprised to find that your body acts quite differently if its fuel is carbohydrates rather than fats. Let's take a look.

Standard high-carbohydrate diet

Everyone fasts, intentionally or not, during sleep. There is no one standard for the length of time required to claim you have "fasted," but studies show that fasting for at least 12 hours at a time (and even better, 16 or 24 hours) is useful for a host of reasons, like a long life and freedom from chronic health problems such as cancer and diabetes. This benefit is likely related to a process called *autophagy,* which occurs when you stop eating and helps to "clean up" and repair the cells of your body.

During this time, the body still has enough stored glycogen to use as a reserve for fuel. *Remember:* Most people eating a diet high in carbohydrates have at least a day's worth of glycogen stored in the liver and muscle, a source of quickly available glucose when it's needed. People who fast overnight or even do intermittent fasting for 16 hours or more won't enter ketosis, even though they do get the benefits associated with autophagy. It takes several days of fasting from a high-carbohydrate diet to move you into ketosis.

Generally, fasting for high-carb dieters will lead to a slight rise in ketones, but not nearly enough to make the body shift toward using ketones as the primary source of energy. That's why people tend to have the highest level of ketones in their urine when they first wake up in the morning.

Keto diet

Some people on the keto diet intermittently fast as well, fueling their ketosis even more. Because someone on the keto diet is always in ketosis, intermittent fasting will allow him or her to go more deeply into the process and reap even more benefits than the high-carb dieter.

As you fast on the keto diet, your body has to use its stores of fat, rather than what you just ate, to fuel itself, which will help you lose even more weight and fat faster than when you eat three times a day on the keto diet. A recent study showed that combining a low-carbohydrate diet and intermittent fasting caused increased weight loss and improved insulin levels, compared to calorie restriction alone. The keto diet may enhance autophagy; not only is it promoted by fasting but it's also induced by restricting carbohydrates, suggesting that keto dieters gain more benefits from intermittent fasting than someone on a high-carb diet.

TIP

Combining the keto diet and intermittent fasting can take you to the next level of your weight loss journey. It also may help keep you healthier as you live longer by combining the benefits of ketones with autophagy, the body's smart way of healing itself.

When the body is in starvation mode

Finally, let's look at starvation. Ketosis isn't starvation in any way, but it's helpful to understand what effect starvation has on the body and how humans have adapted from an evolutionary perspective to combat these effects. In this state, both high-carbohydrate and keto diets start to look a lot alike.

Standard high-carbohydrate diet

After a few days without food, even a high-carbohydrate dieter will enter ketosis because the body isn't getting any new nutrition, so it transitions to the body's stores of energy — fat. Ketone levels rise to the level found in ketosis as they become the primary source of energy. The primary difference between starvation and ketosis is that, in the former, you aren't consuming any new food, while in the latter, you're continuing to eat. This affects your metabolism: When you hit ketosis and you aren't eating anything, hormonal signals trigger a metabolic slowdown. Your brain knows that you're starving and wants to conserve every single calorie it can, meaning it's going to do everything possible to keep you from losing weight.

When you're intentionally in ketosis and still eating, however, your metabolism will continue at the same rate but the body will begin burning excess fat. Maintaining a consistent caloric intake while on the ketogenic diet is what keeps your body from seeing ketosis as starvation.

By the way, this is the reason that so many people who cut down drastically on calories often see plateaus in their weight loss. Their bodies are doing all they can to hold on to the resources they have because, in this state, the body thinks it's starving.

After a long period, or if you've used up your body's fat stores, proteins become the primary source of fuel. As mentioned earlier, this is less than ideal, because it means your muscles and eventually your organs are being broken down to keep you alive. Key processes in the body will come to a halt with prolonged starvation (generally about two weeks, although the amount of time varies from one person to the next) unless you begin to eat again.

Keto diet

Starvation is pretty similar between keto and high-carb dieters. One difference may be your body's ability to adapt to starvation. Because ketosis already mimics starvation with its preference for ketones, your body will not react to deprivation as such a shock to the system. Nevertheless, the same ultimate effect will occur, with the body shutting down as key processes come to a halt.

Anticipating Changes in How You'll Feel

If you're seriously considering starting the keto journey, you're wise to prepare yourself for the changes that lie ahead. This means growth — and sometimes there can be a few growing pains along the way. Just like any adventure, however, there are tons of benefits of going keto, even if there are some hiccups. In this section, we talk about what to expect on the journey.

Short-term changes

Adapting to the keto diet is different for everyone. Drastically cutting out sugar and carbohydrates can be a big shock to the system, but some people don't notice any real changes in the way they feel over the first week or so of adopting a keto lifestyle.

However, some people notice the dreaded keto flu, which happens as your body tries to adapt to a drop in insulin and glucose levels. Keto flu can lead to dehydration and low potassium levels if you aren't careful.

Common symptoms of the keto flu include

>> Dizziness and headaches

>> Diarrhea or constipation

>> Fatigue and feeling weak

>> Flu-like symptoms

>> Muscle cramps

>> Stomach pain

>> Sugar cravings

TIP

A simple way to combat these changes is to drink more water and add salt and potassium into your diet. An additional hack is to take magnesium; potassium losses can lead to muscle cramps, which magnesium helps reduce.

REMEMBER

The keto flu usually lasts less than a week. If you stay hydrated and make sure you aren't losing essential electrolytes, it's likely you won't encounter it at all.

As we mention in Chapter 2, keto breath is another short-term change that sometimes happens as you change to a keto diet. This fruity smelling breath can be bothersome if you happen to get it, but it's only temporary. To combat it, be extra diligent about your oral hygiene and drink more water until it subsides.

Long-term changes

After being on a keto diet for a long time, we've noticed that as much as we enjoy traveling and having extra cheat days (local cuisine is a must-have anywhere new that we go, and most of the time it involves plenty of carbs), we crave coming home and getting back into our keto lifestyle. There's nothing like having consistent, high energy levels every day, and we're reminded of how different life was before keto when we travel.

Many people feel just like us. There are so many benefits of the keto diet, like increased energy and a clear and focused mind, that you'll think twice about "cheating." You'll soon easily tell when you're not in ketosis and notice you don't feel at your best. Also, if you have some weight to lose, the rapid weight loss will be a strong motivation to keep going.

Over time, we've noticed that we don't crave pasta or bread and, believe it or not, sugary treats like ice cream and cake seem almost too much to bear. Your taste buds will change on the keto diet, and you won't have all-consuming cravings.

Some people find that they're constipated on the keto diet. Constipation is not specific to the keto diet, but as you're figuring out what you can and can't eat, you might unintentionally avoid keto-friendly foods high in fiber (like walnuts) or that combat constipation (like MCT oils). Some people choose to add a high-quality fiber supplement, but you can keep up with your fiber needs by eating a well-balanced diet and staying hydrated.

Your blood glucose on a keto diet won't spike. Here is where the benefits of the keto diet are the most evident — by controlling your body's insulin response, you're in full control of your health and your weight. It's an incredibly liberating feeling not to wonder continually, "When's my next meal?"

TIP

The keto lifestyle is a long-term healthy lifestyle. Over time, you'll feel great and barely miss the carbs you once thought you couldn't live without.

Testing to See if You're in Ketosis

Knowing if you're in ketosis helps you understand whether what you're eating is correct and will give you confidence that you're doing things correctly. It's a great feeling to know that you're on track to lose weight, become healthier, and reap all the other benefits of the keto diet.

The good news is that you can begin checking whether ketosis is taking place in your body only three days after starting the diet. Testing for ketosis can be done with the help of a few products.

Urinalysis testing

Ketone urinalysis test strips can help you quickly determine whether you're in ketosis by testing for the presence of excess ketone bodies in your urine. The strips have a small pad which is dipped in a fresh urine specimen and changes color within a few seconds.

Here's how to perform a urine ketone test:

1. **Remove a test strip from the bottle and close the container immediately.**

2. **While holding the end of the strip farthest away from the test pad, pass the test pad through your urine stream.**

   If you prefer, you can collect your urine in a clean, dry container for testing. After collection, quickly dip the test pad into the urine. Drag the long edge of the test strip against the rim of the cup to remove excess urine.

3. **After 15 seconds, match the test pad to the color chart on the label on the bottle of test strips.**

   Color chart blocks give approximate values; actual colors may be slightly darker or lighter than the color shown on the chart.

4. **Discard the used test strip.**

Depending on the levels of ketone bodies in the urine, the pad will change from gray/beige (negative) to a deep purple (high level of ketone bodies). Any shade of purple indicates that you're in ketosis. If you're trying to check your ketones daily, try to stick to a specific time of day, ideally in the morning or several hours after your last meal for the best comparison.

You can purchase ketone testing strips over-the-counter at a local pharmacy, as well as online. Each bottle usually contains 100 to 200 test strips. Although urine test strips are relatively inexpensive (about 5 to 10 cents per strip), they're also much less accurate than blood ketone meters.

Blood testing

Ketone blood test meters are another way to determine if you're in ketosis by directly measuring your blood's β-hydroxybutyrate ketone levels.

Here's how a blood ketone test works:

1. **Wash your hands with soap and dry them.**

2. **Load a needle into the lancet, according to the directions provided.**

3. **Insert a test strip into the meter.**

4. **Place the lancet pen on your fingertip and push the button to draw a small drop of blood.**

5. **Touch the strip to the drop of blood until it fills the opening.**

6. **Check the meter for the reading and compare it to the legend provided.**

    Results between 0.5 and 3 mmol/L indicate that you're in nutritional ketosis.

7. **Dispose of the strip and lancet per the instructions provided.**

You can purchase ketone blood meters and strips at most pharmacies, as well as online. Blood strips usually cost about $1 per strip but also require a blood ketone meter, which can cost upwards of $80 (although it's just a one-time purchase). Testing your blood is much more reliable and accurate than testing your urine.

Chapter **4**

Getting to Know Your Macros

The keto diet is a high-fat, moderate-protein, and very-low-carbohydrate lifestyle. There are clear guidelines on how much, or how little, of each macronutrient you should eat to shift your body into ketosis. Getting familiar with these three macros is crucial so you can quickly learn how to thrive on the keto diet. As you begin the keto diet, you'll learn the value of reading nutrition labels — not just superficially scanning the overall calories, but reviewing the sum total of macros in each serving. In this chapter, we give you a head start on becoming a pro at choosing what to eat.

Loading Up on Healthy Fats

Just like a "calorie is not at a calorie," all fats are not created equal. For example, there are four naturally occurring fats that you typically notice on nutrition labels:

» Saturated

» Monounsaturated

>> Polyunsaturated (this includes omega 3s)

>> Cholesterol (technically, this is more a cousin of fat, but will into more detail about that later in this section)

Research shows that the human body uses these four groups of fats quite differently. You need all of them to function correctly, but some people get too much of certain kinds and not enough of others. Here are the different types of fats, as well as which (and how much) you should be eating.

Healthy fats

You need all four types of fats as part of a well-rounded keto diet, but there are certain fats that you should continuously reach for. The two fats that have the best track record are monounsaturated fats and the omega-3 fatty acids (which are part of the polyunsaturated family).

Monounsaturated fatty acids

You've probably heard about the heart health and long life enjoyed in Mediterranean countries. The Mediterranean diet put olive oil on the map. Talk to any nutritionist, and she'll tell you that olive oil should be the primary oil you eat. The key to olive oil's heart-promoting health is that its fat content is over 70 percent monounsaturated fatty acids (MUFAs). Not only do MUFAs decrease low-density lipoprotein (LDL) cholesterol (the bad kind), but they may even raise high-density lipoprotein (HDL) cholesterol (the good kind). Saturated fats and carbohydrates do the opposite.

In sum, MUFAs:

>> Decrease the risk of getting diabetes.

>> Improve blood pressure control.

>> Decrease inflammation in the arteries, a leading cause of heart disease.

Without a doubt, a diet high in MUFAs is better than a low-fat diet in people who are at risk for heart disease. It helps decrease the risk of future heart attacks and strokes. Some nutritionists are starting to realize that MUFAs are so good for our hearts that they're throwing away the idea that a low-fat, complex-carb diet is best for people with diabetes and asking them to increase their MUFAs instead.

REMEMBER

MUFAs are also plentiful in many animal foods like meat and dairy products. However, several studies that looked at people consuming MUFAs primarily from animal foods did not show the same benefits as people who got their MUFAs from olive oil. The moral? It matters where your fat comes from.

Despite all the benefits that MUFAs offer, the American Heart Association (AHA) tells Americans to limit MUFAs to 15 percent to 20 percent. You'll be reaching for these healthy fats a lot more often on the keto diet.

TIP

Did you know that high-oleic sunflower oil has even more MUFAs than olive oil? It comes in at a whopping 85.4 percent (compared to 73 percent for olive oil). High-oleic sunflower oil is a good option to add to your pantry as you switch to keto.

Omega-3 fatty acids

Another fat that offers benefits for heart health is the omega-3 family. You've probably walked by an aisle full of fish oil tablets and wondered if you should start popping these pills daily. There is a reason for the hype: Omega-3s are anti-inflammatory powerhouses, decreasing the risk of heart disease and possibly a host of other inflammatory conditions, such as Alzheimer's disease.

They aren't all made equally, however. (We hope you're catching on to the recurring theme here!) The two types that are good for you are eicosapentaenoic acid (EPA) and docosahexaenoic acid (DHA), which are found in fatty fish like salmon and anchovies, as well as seaweed and algae.

The third type of omega-3 — alpha-linolenic acid (ALA) — isn't so heart-healthy. That's because the body needs to turn ALA into either EPA or DHA, and it's just not very good at completing that task. You'd have to eat about six times as much ALA-rich foods to get the same benefit from eating EPA- and DHA-rich salmon.

Luckily, you won't waste your time looking for omega-3s in ALA-rich foods on the keto diet. ALAs are primarily found in less healthy vegetable oils and dense carbohydrate foods like grains. If you see a vegetable oil claiming that it has omega-3, it's likely ALA and not worth your time. Even healthy, keto-friendly foods, like flaxseed, chia seed, and walnuts (which are still very good for you), should not be your primary source of omega-3s because they primarily contain ALA.

The recommended goal for omega-3s is between 1 and 3 grams per day to maintain a healthy heart.

TIP

Did you know that you can get algae oil supplements, as an alternative to fish oil supplements? If you're a vegan, this option may appeal to you. Just make sure that if you choose a supplement, it clearly states how much EPA and DHA it contains.

Less healthy fats

Now that you know the powerhouses of fats, let's take a look at fats you can still enjoy, but not quite as often. You'll likely eat these fats every day on the keto diet, but make sure you aren't getting the majority of your fat calories from them.

Saturated fats

There's quite a bit of bad press around saturated fat. It has been demonized by most nutritionists and cardiologists as terrible for your heart. The AHA recommends that people get only 10 percent of their calories from saturated fat. The organization points to higher levels of heart disease, higher LDL, and lower HDL in people who eat more than their recommended levels of saturated fat.

However, there has been a recent backlash to this guidance. Newer research is showing that saturated fat and heart disease are not so tightly linked. Populations of people who ate higher-than-recommended levels of saturated fat were not always more likely to have heart attacks, strokes, or other signs of heart disease. Moreover, compared to the carbohydrates most Americans are eating — bread, potatoes, and pasta — saturated fat may improve your heart health. Research shows that refined carbohydrate-rich diets may be more likely to cause heart disease than saturated fats.

Another boon to the cause for saturated fat is the increasing popularity of coconut oil, which comes in at a whopping 90 percent saturated fat. It's a little different from other saturated fat because it's a rare example of a plant-based saturated fat; most of the saturated fat people eat is from meat or dairy products. Coconut oil is made up of different types of saturated fats as well: It's high in medium-chain fats that the body absorbs quickly and burns for fuel (as compared to long-chain fats found in animal foods). Long-chain fats are more likely to be stored as fat when you overindulge.

Eating too much saturated fat in the context of a high-carbohydrate diet — think a classic cheeseburger with fries on the side — is a dangerous combination. Within the keto diet, you're probably going to increase the amount of saturated fat you eat as your overall calories from fat increase. But consuming saturated fat within a whole foods diet, with a wide range of healthy fats and low, fiber-rich carbs, is hardly the death sentence that some cardiologists would have you believe.

TIP

Saturated fat is not all bad. Recent research shows that eating saturated fat is better for you than eating excess carbs.

Cholesterol

Cholesterol also gets a bad rap from conventional nutritional wisdom, but it, too, has been vilified unfairly. Eating high-cholesterol foods does not translate into high cholesterol levels in the way you might think. What you eat matters, but the human body is more complicated than people give it credit for. The liver is capable of making all the cholesterol you need, without having to turn to cholesterol-rich foods. Plus, you need cholesterol to survive — it's a vital player in the body as

>> A building block of many hormones

>> An integral part of cell membranes

>> An ingredient of "fat-soluble" vitamins, like A, D, E and K

>> A necessary component that helps to digest food

What you think of as your "cholesterol" level is made up of lipoproteins like LDL and HDL. These lipoproteins are the molecules that shuttle cholesterol around in the blood, rather than the cholesterol that does the critical work in the body. Although some of these lipoproteins increase heart disease, there is a lot of misinformation about which ones.

Although doctors always thought of LDL as "bad" cholesterol, it's really not that simple. There are several types of LDL, and some don't deserve the moniker "bad." Small, dense LDL is the "bad" stuff, which derails heart health, while the larger, fluffier LDL is more like HDL, and may eventually be classified differently than other types of LDL.

The important part is that lipoproteins are affected by the types of non-cholesterol foods you eat. LDL rises when you eat trans fats, simple carbohydrates, and excessive saturated fats, but the amount of cholesterol you eat doesn't affect it significantly. It's vital to look at the range of nutrients in your food, rather than mindlessly cut out all cholesterol.

Where you get your cholesterol matters: There are some foods with high levels of cholesterol that come with a host of benefits, making them healthy choices for a whole-food keto diet. For example, egg yolks are high in cholesterol but come packed with essential nutrients, like choline, vitamins A and D, zinc, calcium, iron, selenium, and omega-3s, to name a few. Eggs are a nutrient-rich food that you shouldn't overlook.

The AHA recently changed its recommendation that people eat only 300 milligrams of cholesterol per day, which is about one-and-a-half eggs. That's because research consistently demonstrates that eating cholesterol doesn't worsen cholesterol. The guidelines still suggest that people should "limit" high-cholesterol foods (although they don't specify an upper limit) because they're often high in saturated fat, but the massive change in thinking about cholesterol is a harbinger that it's just a matter of time before the recommendations regarding saturated fat are changed.

Cholesterol is not the villain it has been made out to be. Your "cholesterol" levels have very little to do with the amount of dietary cholesterol you consumer and more to do with "bad" fats and carbohydrates.

Polyunsaturated fatty acids

Polyunsaturated fatty acids (PUFAs), excluding the omega-3s that we discuss earlier, are on the opposite end of the spectrum from saturated fats. In the same way that many doctors currently believe that saturated fats are entirely bad, scientists once thought that PUFAs were unequivocally good for people, but research is showing that they may have some hidden drawbacks. This other group of PUFAs is called omega-6s (compared to the heart-healthy omega-3s).

Currently, the AHA recommends that 5 percent to 10 percent of a person's calories come from omega-6 fats. However, PUFAs are found in a wide range of foods — from vegetable oils, like soybean oil, to walnuts and fatty fish — so very few people don't get enough. Conventionally, people have been taught that PUFAs are healthier than saturated fats and should be chosen over them.

However, it's not quite that simple. Linoleic acid, a common omega-6 PUFA found in vegetable oils, may not be that good for you. Not only does it show no benefit regarding heart disease and stroke, but a study looking at people who were told to choose linoleic fat instead of saturated fat found that they were more likely to die from heart disease and heart attacks. Because Americans often get these fats from dubious sources, like soybean oil and corn oil, the most common cooking oils in American pantries, this is quite concerning.

There is a silver lining for keto dieters. Conjugated linoleic acid, which is commonly found in organically raised beef and dairy products, is good for you. Studies show that these type of omega-6 fats may have a hand in reducing the risk of cancer, diabetes, and heart disease. Here, the source of the food matters, and in the case of linoleic acid, organic animal foods trump processed vegetable foods.

Still, compared to omega-3s, omega-6 fats tend to increase inflammation. And increasing inflammation is associated with the most common long-term health problems in our society: heart disease, cancer, and autoimmune disease.

When you shift your consumption too far to the omega-6 side, you actually stop your body's ability to benefit from the anti-inflammatory advantages of omega-3s. This is because the body uses the same metabolic pathways for all PUFAs, regardless of whether they increase or decrease inflammation. Overeating omega-6s not only increases inflammation in the body, but it also blocks your body's ability to heal by using EPA and DHA. Americans eat about 15 times more omega-6s than omega-3s, whereas our ancestors probably consumed an equal amount of both. That's a huge change that's showing up as the common health problems so many of us struggle with.

Most nutrition labels aren't going to tell you the ratio of omega-3s to other PUFAs so you may have to do a little more digging to uncover the types of PUFAs you're eating. Generally, cooking oils like soybean oil and corn oil are going to have much more omega-6s than walnuts or flaxseed oils (which also have ALA).

Another thing about PUFA oils is that they tend to *oxidize* (go bad) quickly if you leave them out too long. They also shouldn't be used as cooking oils because they have a lower smoke point and lose all their health benefits when overheated. Many PUFA oils need to be put in the refrigerator in a dark container and thrown out immediately if they start smelling funny.

REMEMBER

The source of your PUFAs matters. Although the PUFAs found in dubious vegetable oils can increase inflammation and chronic diseases, high-quality PUFAs in organic beef and dairy can prevent these risks and help you thrive on the keto lifestyle.

Unhealthy fats

Now that we've talked about what you *should* be eating, let's talk about the fats that are entirely unhealthy and should have no part in a healthy keto diet: trans fats. Just say no to them!

There are small amounts of natural trans fats found in animal meat and dairy products that are fine to eat. Beyond this, however, everyone can agree that you should stay far away from human-made trans fats. Food scientists made these unnatural oils in laboratories to allow food to remain edible longer (to be transported thousands of miles or stay on a grocery shelf for months on end). That's why these fats are high in packaged goods like Twinkies.

More and more customers are aware of the problems associated with trans fats — they increase the risk of heart disease — and stay away from any food that lists trans fat on the nutrition label. However, food manufacturers are sneaky: They can label their foods as "trans-fat free," but add up to half a gram per serving, which means that if you eat enough these "trans-fat free" foods, you may start to have quite a bit of trans fats in your diet. Hidden trans fats are sometimes labeled "partially hydrogenated" oils, so make sure to turn down any food that has this in the ingredient list. Luckily, trans fats are typically in preserved junk food that is off limits on the keto diet.

It's a pretty common misconception that the keto diet is a high-protein lifestyle. Let's be clear: Keto is not high protein. Protein is vital in the keto lifestyle, but you should only be eating moderate amounts, or just as much as your body needs. Generally, the goal is 0.36 gram per pound of body weight in the person who is moderately active, although high-level athletes can go up to 0.8 grams per pound and a very sedentary person should probably eat a little less than 0.36 gram per pound of body weight.

Consuming Moderate Amounts of Protein

Overeating protein can derail your ketosis. Proteins cause a spike in insulin levels. So, even if there is no glucose in your diet, excess protein can be used by the body to make glucose through the gluconeogenesis process. That means that if you choose to eat more protein than your body needs, you could push yourself out of ketosis and go back to wild highs and lows of glucose and insulin spikes.

REMEMBER

Be aware of the range of protein available to you in the keto lifestyle and approximately how much you need to support your muscles, organs, and essential body processes while keeping yourself in ketosis. Not only are your protein sources vital, but where you get them is also critical. You need to know what a serving size is and which veggie and animal foods are ideal sources of protein.

Cutting Unnecessary Carb Consumption

Beyond a bare minimum, carbs are not necessary for your survival, despite what the U.S. Department of Agriculture (USDA) "Choose My Plate" approach recommends — which, ironically, has no place on your plate for fat at all! — or what well-meaning friends say. As we explain in Chapter 3, your liver is quite capable of making all the glucose your body needs without any help from the bread basket. The benefit of going keto is that you're cutting out carbs that are found in unhealthy prepackaged food that humans have only been eating for a relatively short time. It's like going back a hundred years or so when convenient and unhealthy breakfast cereals, pasta, and bread were not the norm. Our grandparents and great-grandparents could not easily munch on bagels and granola bars as they went to work, and instead ate higher-fat, lower-carb foods and stayed slimmer than we do today.

The keto diet allows you to let go of the cravings that have kept you tied down to high-carb foods. Carbs often leave you feeling sluggish and bloated when you indulge, leading to a love-hate relationship. By cutting your carbs to only 5 percent of your intake, you'll rid yourself of the uncomfortable feelings associated with carbs and feel more energized throughout the day. Also, in a world that is increasingly keto-friendly, you'll be able to find other highly nutritious foods to fuel your body. Going low-carb will open your diet up to vegetables you may have overlooked. Some of our favorite keto-friendly carbs are:

>> Zucchini

>> Cauliflower

>> Brussels sprouts

>> Mushrooms

>> Red bell peppers

Not only are these low in carbs, but they also have a built-in host of minerals, vitamins, and antioxidants that will leave you feeling great. With a little know-how and a couple of the recipes in Part 5 of this book, you'll be eating these wonder veggies regularly!

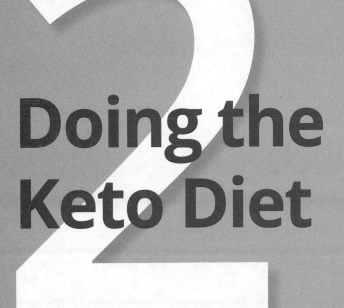

2
Doing the Keto Diet

Chapter **5**

Stocking Up on Keto-Friendly Foods

I n this chapter, we tell you what to eat and what to stay far away from on the keto diet. You'll need to take a critical look at your fridge, pantry, and that little snack drawer in your car, office, or wherever you hide it. We show you how to clear out carb-heavy foods and replace them with healthy, whole-food keto items to keep you satisfied for hours to come.

Keto goes back to what your body knows: Fat is good for you, and carbs are not a necessary nutrient. As you start the keto journey, you'll need to do a complete mind — and pantry — makeover. As you let go of the false nutrition claims that you've ingested over the years, you'll more easily rid your cupboards of all the low-fat foods you thought were healthy, and instead turn to filling, delicious, good-for-you foods that will nourish your body and mind.

REMEMBER

You're not sacrificing flavor to go keto. In fact, one of the hallmarks of this diet is its abundant offerings for your taste buds. Fat is nature's flavoring, and you get full access to its entire spectrum. Because the Western world is so centered around carbs and excess sugar, it may take some time for your taste buds to recover from the sweetness overstimulation they've been subjected to for years, but when that adjustment takes place, you'll find an unparalleled gourmet dining experience waiting for you.

Out with the Old: Clearing Out Your Carb-Heavy Stock

If you're like most Americans, you've probably got pantry shelves filled with carb-heavy staples — flour, bread, rice, sugar, and other items that are your default ingredients for all your meals, from a quick lunch on the go to a beautiful five-course anniversary dinner. Be aware that these staples have no place in a keto-friendly kitchen. Not to worry! We're here to show you how to get rid of these items that will derail you from your ketogenic journey.

TIP

If you're part of a "mixed" household — where some members of the home are on keto and others are not — things are a bit more complicated because you won't be able to eliminate as many temptations outright, but there are specific steps you can take to bolster your chances of success.

>> **Reorganize your drawers, cupboards, and cabinets.** Label each drawer or cabinet either "keto" or "the devil" (we're just kidding — you're probably safer going with "non-keto"), and divide your foods accordingly. This will help when you experience cravings, or open a door and you're unexpectedly staring face-to-face with all the ingredients necessary to make your favorite cake.

>> **Cook and eat your food first — especially if you're going to be the one making both a non-keto meal and a keto one.** We all know that it's a bad idea to go to the grocery store when we're hungry, and the same principle applies to cooking non-keto while on keto. You should eat first; then enter regular meal prep in a satiated state.

>> **Introduce keto meals to your non-keto family, friends, and roommates.** Keep track of the ones they like, and then slowly rotate them into the regular meals. Even if you don't convince the people living with you to give keto a try, the more food you can put on the table that aligns with your macros, the lower your temptation will be every time a meal is served.

>> **If you're going to do intermittent fasting, think through your family's typical eating schedule and how your feeding window will match up with that.** Let's say, for example, that you've got to make breakfast for your family and get your kids off to school, but your feeding window is from 12 p.m. to 8 p.m. By the time breakfast rolls around, you may not have eaten for 12 hours, and you've got another 4 to go before you can do anything about it — and now you're making pancakes.

Consider shifting your feeding window to an earlier time. Feel free to play around with it. There are no hard and fast rules to intermittent fasting — they're more just guidelines, and you can customize every aspect of it to your specific situation. Because you can have coffee and tea, you might consider having a large cup before you start cooking because these drinks can take the edge off your hunger.

If you're someone who doesn't like breakfast anyway, this might be a non-issue. However, at some point, you're going to run into situations where intermittent fasting just doesn't line up well with your life, and going through this exercise is very useful.

In the following sections, we walk you through what to eliminate from your keto-friendly kitchen (or at least the portion of the kitchen where you store your keto-friendly foods).

Ridding your shelves of sugar

Sugar is the real reason you can't shed unwanted pounds, and you're still carrying around that irritating muffin top. As the sugars you eat drive your insulin levels up and direct your body to store excess fat, you put yourself in an uphill battle to maintain a healthy weight — or fit into your favorite jeans from your high school days. Cutting excess sugar out of your life is the first step toward reversing this problem.

Sugar has a very high glycemic index (GI) and causes a rapid spike in insulin. This sweet substance can cause a dramatic increase in inflammation and irritation in your body, leading to brain fog, headaches, and a host of other issues. The associated high levels of insulin not only increase your storage of fat, but also increase the risk for other serious diseases like heart disease, high blood pressure, liver disease, and even problems with fertility.

You may be thinking: What about alternative sugars like honey, coconut sugar, and dates? Aren't they healthy alternatives with antioxidants, micronutrients, fiber, and even antibacterial properties? Yes, these sugars may come with benefits lacking in white granulated sugar, but regardless of this potential benefit, they're all, at their core, sugar. Honey has more grams of carbs per serving than table sugar. All these sweeteners are high on the GI for food, meaning they can all contribute to your risk of developing diabetes, heart disease, and a host of other conditions. Just say no to all sugars.

Here are the sugars that you must ditch from your pantry (whether they're standalone products or part of packaged foods):

>> **Brown, white, or turbinado sugar:** These are all products from sugarcane and are high in calories and carbs. The differences between them are minuscule — turbinado sugar is slightly less processed than brown or white

sugar, but they're all essentially empty carbs. Turbinado and brown sugar have small amounts of your daily iron intake (from the molasses content) and nothing else. White sugar is not only processed, but also bleached and may have chemical residues that harm your health. These are a waste of calories, and there are plenty of approved artificial sweeteners you can use instead. Avoid brown, white, and turbinado sugar at all costs.

>> **Sucanat:** This is one of the least-processed forms of sugarcane. Don't let that fool you into thinking it's healthy, though. Sucanat is still a high-GI food with only minute amounts of minerals and just as many carbs and calories as highly processed white sugar. It will kick you out of ketosis just like any other sugar product will. Similar products may go by the name of muscovado, khand (India), jaggery (South Asia), and panela (Latin America), depending on what part of the world you find yourself in.

>> **Coconut sugar:** Made from the coconut palm tree, rather than sugarcane, coconut sugar is touted as a healthy alternative because it may have a slightly lower GI than other sugars. Again, though it has some trace nutrients and even a bit of fiber, it has just as many empty calories as refined white sugar and will still cause a spike in your blood sugar when you use it. This sweetener isn't worth your time.

>> **Honey:** Produced from the honeybee's reprocessing of flower nectar, honey does have some benefits, such as its anti-inflammatory and antioxidant properties. However, it has even more calories than sugar does and still spikes your blood sugar levels. We think it's best to use honey as a face mask, where you can reap all the benefits without causing excess weight gain. ***Remember:*** You can get the nutrients in honey elsewhere, but without the sugars.

>> **Molasses:** This product of sugarcane is what gives brown sugar its color. It's less processed than brown sugar and provides virtually the same nutritional value of any form of sugar. Although it can be a good source of potassium and certain minerals, it is still 75 percent sugar (the rest is water and trace minerals), so it has no place on the keto diet. You can easily get more minerals from a number of healthy keto foods that won't shoot your blood sugar through the roof.

>> **Agave:** Although considered a "natural" alternative to sugar, agave is primarily made of fructose, the other sugar molecule that can cause worse effects on your body when combined with glucose. Because it has a sugar mix similar to high-fructose corn syrup, it should be used very sparingly. High levels of fructose can cause liver damage and increase weight gain, even more so than high levels of glucose. This option may even be worse than white sugar for your health over the long term. We recommend that you avoid anything that uses this as a sweetener. Luckily, you can still enjoy tequila — although it also comes from agave, all the fructose from the plant has already been distilled away.

>> **Dates:** Another "natural" and better-for-you sugar, dates are still are made up of about 80 percent sugar. They come with fiber and some vitamins, but just three dates provide about 50 grams of sugar. You can see how it would be easy to be kicked out of ketosis if you kept any of these on hand. Dates are an excellent example of an all-natural, even organic source of sugar that you still have to avoid.

>> **Syrups:** This includes maple syrup, corn syrup, and rice varieties. These are all essentially sugar water.

TIP

Set aside a couple of hours one day and go through every item in your kitchen, refrigerator, and pantry. Check out the nutrition labels and divide everything into keto-approved and non-keto-approved piles. This may be one of the most educational activities you'll ever experience — we guarantee you'll be shocked at the places you find significant amounts of carbs. Sausage, salsa, flavored milk alternatives (soy, rice, almond, and so on), and even certain types of bacon (we know, you probably thought any kind of bacon was keto-approved — so did we, at first) can be loaded with sugar. Reading the labels will help you get a firm grasp on how pervasive sugar is in every aspect of our diets.

REMEMBER

Ingredient lists rarely state something as simple as "sugar." There are several alternate names for sugar you should be aware of. Scan the nutrition labels and toss foods with any of these:

>> Maltodextrin

>> Fruit juice concentrate

>> Cane sugar

>> Dextrose

>> Sucrose

>> Saccharose

>> High-fructose corn syrup

>> Glucose-fructose syrup

WARNING

Be wary of most artificial sugars. Although these no-calorie sweeteners tout their lack of carbs, your body can still be tricked into thinking they're sugar and release insulin. When you eat something sweet, whether it's artificial or not, the sweet receptors on your tongue can trigger a set of reactions that tells your body to prepare for a carbohydrate load. While artificial sweeteners are designed to avoid raising blood sugar levels, some studies have shown that certain sweeteners, like sucralose and acesulfame potassium, can trigger spikes in insulin, even without calories or carbs. Due to these effects on insulin, they can cause similar problems of weight gain, diabetes, and heart disease that comes along with levels of insulin in the blood that are too high.

Even apart from spiking insulin levels, these "sugar substitutes" can continue your addiction to the sweet taste and keep you chained to sweetened foods, many of which are often packaged and processed, even if they are "keto friendly." *Remember:* The goal is to avoid raising your blood sugar and triggering an insulin spike, which can be caused by foods that are otherwise "good."

Artificial sweeteners include

>> Aspartame (NutraSweet)

>> Sucralose (Splenda)

>> Saccharin (Sweet'N Low)

>> Acesulfame potassium (Ace-K, Sunette)

>> Mixed artificial sweeteners (Equal)

It's okay to have a dessert once in a while (even on keto). So, later in this chapter, we tell you about the low-GI sugars that you can indulge in occasionally on the keto diet.

Ditching flours and grains

Flours and grains are everywhere, but they have no place in the keto diet. Although not as "simple" as the sugars we mention in the preceding section, these foods will eventually be broken down into their sugar components — and that's just how your body will treat them. Although flour and grain foods have a range of values on the GI, by their very nature carbs will cause your insulin levels to increase, so it's best to stay away from all of them.

Some of these foods, especially the whole-grain varieties, may have some useful nutrients, but there are many keto-friendly foods with the same nutrients — you don't have to get them from carbohydrate sources. It's easy to get wrapped up in the story that whole grains are good for you, but whole grain or not, your body will eventually treat grain as sugar. The truth is, if you look at many whole-wheat foods next to their "white" or refined counterparts, there isn't much of a difference. For example, the GI of white bread is 75, while that of whole-wheat bread is 74. Similarly, white rice's GI is 73, while brown rice has a GI of 68.

When you take into account the variety of different brands, there is no difference at all — these are all high-GI foods and the label "whole-wheat" can't change that fact. It may feel good to choose the whole-grain options, but your body doesn't know the difference and will still have to chase down the whole grains with an unhealthy dose of insulin.

Besides, more people are beginning to realize that they have allergies or food sensitivities to *gluten* (a protein found in wheat, barley, and rye products) and other grains. Gluten is likely a culprit in the increasingly common inflammatory gut conditions. You may have heard of *leaky gut syndrome,* a condition in which your gut lining becomes "leaky" and toxins, bacteria, and other harmful substances bypass normal digestion and are absorbed through intercellular cracks in your gut. Some studies suggest that gluten may encourage breaks in your gut's lining and lead to a host of problems like celiac disease and autoimmune conditions like type 1 diabetes. If you continue to eat lots of grains, with their increasingly higher percentages of gluten and inflammatory sugars, many of which alter your gut flora and lead to intestinal problems, you'll continue to suffer from bloating, brain fog, fatigue, and worse.

Here are the flours and grains to ditch:

>> White and whole-wheat flours (for example, all-purpose, pastry, self-rising)

>> Rice (brown, white, wild)

>> Quinoa

>> Couscous

>> Pasta (such as spaghetti, macaroni, and all noodles)

>> Barley

>> Millet

>> Oats and oatmeal

>> Amaranth

>> Sorghum

>> Teff

>> Triticale

WARNING

Don't be fooled into thinking that all these exotic "ancient" grains are a healthy choice. Even if you could go back to paleo times, it's unlikely that our ancestors were eating these grains several times a day — even if they could find an open fire in a place safe enough to cook them long enough for them to be palatable.

You may have friends and family who object to this list by touting some grains as being packed with nutrition — and they're right. There's no need to argue this point. What they (or at least you) should understand is that every nutrient provided by one of the grains in that list can be found elsewhere, and eating a diet heavy in grains/carbs leads to a host of potential health problems. You're not telling them that whole grains don't have nutrition; you're merely saying that the nutrients you'd gain can be found elsewhere, and you're just replacing the source.

This list also includes all things made up of flours and grains, including bread in its many forms, cereals, tortillas, pastries, pretzels, potato chips, pita, tortilla chips, and many more.

Eliminating starchy vegetables

Starchy vegetables are a high source of carbs. Although vegetables are a nutritional resource on the keto diet, the carbs trump the nutrients for many of them, and those have to go. Often these starchy veggies — like other high-carb foods — can leave you feeling bloated, physically uncomfortable, and mentally unfocused. Because you can find the same nutrients in low-carb vegetables, it's a no-brainer to ditch all the starchy ones.

Here are the vegetables we recommend you ditch:

>> Tubers and root vegetables (such as carrots, potatoes, sweet potatoes, squash, parsnips, and yams)

>> Beans and lentils (including bean-based products like hummus and falafel)

>> Corn

>> Plantains

>> Green peas

>> Pumpkin

>> Corn and cornmeal

Many of these vegetables, even when boiled, are considered high-GI foods. For example, sweet potato's GI of 63 is quite similar to the very sweet pineapple, which is about 59. Don't get fooled into thinking that all veggies are good options for you. Ditch the high-carb vegetables that will raise your blood sugar quickly; regardless of what other redeeming factors they may have, the cost to your blood sugar and insulin levels isn't worth it.

REMEMBER

Another benefit of going keto is that your taste buds will adjust and things that used to taste bland will suddenly become sweeter. You've never truly appreciated how sweet carrots, sweet potatoes, and sweet corn are until you've been on a low-carb diet for an extended period. One of the incredible benefits this creates is that when you want to have something sweet, you're heading for carrots and corn rather than a donut. Even the times you "cheat" won't impact you as much, because you'll be more satisfied with fruits and vegetables that are far better than candy or baked desserts.

Tossing high-glycemic fruits

Most fruits are off-limits on the keto list, but you can have a small amount of approved, keto-friendly fruits once in a while. All fruits contain sugar. Even if it's natural, sugar will still raise your blood glucose and insulin levels, generating unwanted weight along with a potential host of other conditions.

What's more, fruits contain a slightly different sugar, called fructose (as opposed to the glucose that is a primary energy source, if you're not in ketosis). Fructose may be even worse than glucose because it's associated with higher blood sugar levels and a higher risk of diabetes than glucose over the long term. Fructose can't be used directly as an energy source like glucose can; it won't raise your insulin levels immediately, but must first be converted into another substance, such as triglycerides (fat). This is why the sweetener commonly added to processed junk food — high-fructose corn syrup — is so bad for you.

No one is suggesting that an apple is the same as the mega-doses of high-fructose corn syrup found in a can of soda, but the high fructose content found in fruits (and especially fruit juices that don't have the fiber that fruits contain) can contribute to an elevation in blood sugar levels and ultimately fat gain.

Keto uses the GI to divide fruits into keto friendly and unfriendly options This index, which we mention briefly in Chapter 2, is a system that measures a carbohydrate's ability to raise blood sugar levels. The GI scale is rated from 0 to 100, with easily digested and quickly absorbed sugars (like soda) closer to 100 and slowly digested carbs closer to 0. Although the index spans 100 points, no carb ever reaches 0 (only fats and proteins can achieve this).

The importance of the GI is that people who eat a lot of high-GI foods are at increased risk of weight gain, heart disease, strokes, and diabetes. The terms *complex carbohydrate* and *simple sugar* are often used to categorize carbs, but the GI is much more precise and more meaningful.

Here are some common fruits and their respective GIs:

>> **Apples:** 40

>> **Bananas:** 30 to 70 (the riper the banana, the higher the GI)

>> **Kiwi:** 58

>> **Mangoes:** 60

>> **Oranges:** 48

>> **Pineapples:** 59

Too many apples (and especially cups of apple juice) a day may not keep the doctor away after all.

Purging all processed foods

"Packaged food is healthy," said no one ever. All the convenience people seek comes with a high cost, through undiagnosed high blood pressure, diabetes, and heart disease. These foods are made to last a long time on the store shelves, and travel for thousands of miles with a laundry list of preservatives and chemicals to accomplish these goals, all of which can damage your body over time.

As the saying goes, if it has too many syllables and sounds like something out of your high school chemistry textbook, you probably shouldn't be eating it. Common ingredients in packaged food are

>> High-fructose corn syrup

>> Hydrogenated (or partially hydrogenated) oils

>> Soybean, corn, canola, and palm oils

>> Monosodium glutamate

>> Artificial flavors

TIP

One of the general guidelines to use while grocery shopping is that 90 percent of your food should come from the "outer ring." All fresh foods are featured on the exterior walls of the store — the produce, the meat deli, and the refrigerated food section where you'll find meat and dairy products. Most of the food in the center of the store is packaged and processed; little attention needs to be paid to it by the grocer because the expiration dates are measured in months and sometimes years, rather than days. Rid your pantry shelves of these packaged and processed foods and don't buy them again. Your body will thank you, both in the short term and in the long term.

In with the New: Healthy Fats, Proteins, and Carbs

After you rid your pantry shelves and fridge of diabetes-inducing carbs and packaged foods, it's time to fill it up with the good stuff. Get ready for a new way of eating: delicious, filling fats that will leave you satisfied; high-quality protein that will maintain your lean body mass; and an array of nutrient-dense, low-carb veggies.

WHAT *ORGANIC* MEANS

As we introduce you to healthy keto food, eating organic is going to come up, so let's dig into a quick overview of what exactly *organic* means — and doesn't — as well as other commonly seen U.S. Department of Agriculture (USDA) food labeling systems.

Organic foods have no antibiotics, hormones, genetically modified organisms (GMOs), synthetic insecticides, or herbicides, and they require sustainable farming practices. Note that organic foods can still use "natural" herbicides that may pose risks to humans. Also, organic labeling does not say anything about the living condition of the animals. Organic does not translate into "pasture-raised," "free-range," or even "grass-fed." You have to look for these notations on the food you consume to ensure it fulfills these extra requirements.

Importantly, some foods will only be organic to a certain percentage:

- "100 percent organic" means completely organic.
- "Organic foods" are required to be made up of a minimum of 95 percent organic ingredients, but they don't have to be entirely organic.
- "Made with organic ingredients" requires at least 70 percent organic ingredients.

You may also come across "natural" foods. This label is not as rigorously defined but generally indicates that the foods have no artificial ingredients (like food coloring or flavors) and are "minimally" processed.

You've no doubt come across the Non-GMO Project Verified label, which means the food does not contain any genetically modified ingredients. GMOs are ubiquitous — about 75 percent of packaged food has at least one GMO ingredient, and the government requirement for labeling does not reach a grocery store near you until

(continued)

(continued)

at least 2020. Luckily, many food corporations are reluctantly changing their labeling practices ahead of the deadline and will have a statement in microscopic font stating "made with genetically modified ingredient." Still, it's safe to assume that you're eating a GMO product if you buy it packaged in the store that is not organic or does not have the non-GMO Project Verified label.

Why should you care about organic, GMO, and the rest? Controversy exists, but certain organic foods — or at least nonconventional foods — are better for you. Organically raised meat has more omega-3s and less inflammatory polyunsaturated fatty acids (PUFAs) than other choices. The absence of harmful antibiotics and hormones is just as important as the presence of quality nutrients in your food. Cows can be injected with hormones to increase their milk production, and chickens are often given antibiotics to stop them from getting sick and improving yield.

Unfortunately, hormones and antibiotics are transferred to us when we eat these foods, causing unexpected changes in our hormones, or increasing the spread of superbugs that cause infections for which modern medicine has limited treatment options. For vegetables, arguably the most important aspect of organic foods is that they're free from pesticides, which have unsavory health risks and are associated with cancers and other diseases in farm workers and consumers.

The most common GMO crops are corn, soy, cotton, and canola, but there are also fish and nuts that have been modified to reach maturity earlier. The term *GMO* is even more controversial than *organic*. The USDA states that there are no significant differences in nutritional content between GMO and non-GMO, but this may not be entirely accurate. Some proponents say that GMO helps produce food to feed the billions of people calling earth home and is a technology to help combat certain diseases (GMO bananas can produce a hepatitis vaccination!).

However, some of these foods may be a factor in antibiotic resistance, and there are many that we don't know the long-term consequences of regularly consuming. Historically, some of the research has been covered up, leading to a lot of mistrust from consumers.

Throughout this section, we mention when it's worth the extra money to get organic foods and when it's okay to go for conventional food.

Saying hello to healthy fats

Fats are the basis of the keto lifestyle, so get acquainted with them. As you eat an array of different types of fats, you'll wonder why anyone ever chooses to eat low-fat anything! Fat is creamy, rich, and decadent. It's a nutrient of quality and excellent fuel for your life.

Stocking up on eggs

The amazing, edible egg is back! Eggs are a powerhouse of nutrition with an array of fat, protein, and healthy micronutrients. You'll never need to ask for just egg whites on keto; instead, you'll eat the whole egg — yolk included — and thoroughly enjoy it. Eggs were demonized in the past because of the concern of high levels of cholesterol (about 150 mg in a medium-size egg), but this concern has dissipated as scientists realized that dietary cholesterol does not cause high blood cholesterol levels and studies show that eating eggs daily does not increase the risk of heart disease.

Eggs are a major source of choline, which is an essential nutrient in metabolism and is a factor in increasing brain health. It helps produce acetylcholine, a neurotransmitter that's vital for brain development, mood regulation, and improving overall learning and muscle function. Eggs also contain a host of vitamins and minerals, such as anti-inflammatory zinc and selenium.

Eggs can be eaten in many ways and used in a variety of meals. Hard-boiled eggs are a nutritious on-the-go meal while whipping up some eggs and cream into a mini frittata is a wonderful way to fill up on all of an egg's goodness. You'll find some more great ideas in Part 5 of this book.

REMEMBER

When it comes to eggs, quality is critical. Make sure you take a moment to investigate how the chickens that laid your eggs were treated. Environmental factors matter because free-range eggs exposed to sunlight have increased levels of vitamin D in their eggs and those fed omega-3-enriched feed lay eggs richer in omega-3 fats. It's always a great idea to get eggs from a farmer's market, join a community-supported agriculture (CSA) group, or even raise your own chickens, but many people have to get eggs from the grocery store. Organic matters and eggs should be of high quality — especially when they're a go-to food, as they often are on the keto diet.

TIP

We recommend you spend the extra money to get organic, free-range eggs unless you're lucky enough to get your eggs from a local farmer's market or a farmer in your area.

READING THE LABELS ON EGG CARTONS

When it comes to eggs, retailers and producers have created quite a few terms that need to be explained. As you may expect, they're designed to sound far more reassuring than what the term actually means.

- **Omega-3 enriched:** This term means that the chickens were fed a diet that was rich in omega-3s, often in the form of flaxseeds. Theoretically, this is a good thing, but it's also important to know that the Food and Drug Administration (FDA) only regulates this term when there's a complaint against a specific farm. You've likely never independently tested your eggs to see how much omega-3s you were getting, and that's pretty typical. This term doesn't communicate much because there are no real standards producers have to abide by in order to use it.

- **Vegetarian fed:** This term is misleading. It conjures up images of happy chickens being fed a well-balanced diet filled with fresh vegetables and roughage, but this isn't the case. The birds are typically fed a prepared mix of corn and soy, which are not the most nutritious of grains.

- **Cage-free:** Yet another misleading term. This one makes you think of a sea of chickens in a field, free to come and go as they please, only coming inside to roost at night. Unfortunately, the industry takes this one very literally: Instead of packing chickens three-tight in cages, they can still pack them several-hundred tight in a room that can only hold several hundred chickens. Technically speaking, there are no cages, so they're legally allowed to advertise this. As you can imagine, though, the reality is very disappointing when compared to your expectations of what this term meant.

- **Farm-fresh or natural:** These terms have no formal definition, no explicit standards, and no one regulates them. In other words, they mean nothing, and eggs you see labeled this way could be the same eggs that you see two packages over for half the price.

- **Pasture-raised:** This term has meaning. Chickens with this label are allowed to come and go from the outside to the barn. They can forage for worms and small insects, be more selective with their food choices, and get more exercise — all of which are good things when you're making an egg in your body! This is the number one label we recommend you look for when buying eggs.

- **Free-range or free-roaming:** This label is just slightly above *cage-free* in its standards. The birds are kept in large barns and have some freedom of movement; they usually have some access to outside. However, there are no regulations regarding the amount of time the birds are allowed outside, what kind of terrain they're let free on, or any other of a number of crucial factors that directly impact the egg's nutritional development.

- **Certified organic:** The value of this label is debatable, but at least it's well defined. The USDA requires that eggs with this label be laid by chickens who are antibiotic- and pesticide-free, fed an all-vegetarian diet, and have access to the outdoors. The outdoor time and environment are undefined, and a vegetarian diet isn't the best for chickens — they're omnivores, and a crucial source of protein for them is comprised of worms and bugs. However, at least you have some idea what you're getting when you buy a certified organic carton of eggs.

Opting for fattier cuts of meat and poultry

Say no to tasteless, skinless chicken breast and other lackluster lean meats. On keto, you're going for the full-fat cuts of beef. It's okay to have some saturated fat in your diet — saturated fat is not directly linked to heart disease and stroke as some earlier nutritional guidelines suggest — so you can enjoy the best parts of meat. You can add back the higher-fat cuts of beef:

>> Tenderloin

>> Ribeye

>> Porterhouse

>> Flap steak

>> Filet mignon

>> Skirt steak

>> New York strip

>> T-bone

>> Prime rib

>> Pork tenderloin

>> Pork or beef ribs

When you eat these meats, opt for quality. Meats and poultry are affected by their environment — make sure to eat grass-fed beef and antibiotic-free chicken.

REMEMBER

Go outside your comfort zone and seek out wild meats, like bison, pheasant, and duck, for the occasional treat. These animals are often naturally free-range and more likely to be organic, so you can be more confident about their environmental conditions and nutrition quality. Grass-fed beef and free-range meats may be more expensive, but the quality speaks for itself.

TIP

Think about getting more substantial quantities of meat (like the whole chicken, rather than just the thighs or drumsticks) because you can save money by buying the entire animal and easily save the leftovers for a long time in your freezer. Besides, you get the nutrition of the whole animal, including the gelatin and nutrients from the bones that can be used to make a good bone broth later.

REMEMBER

Stick to healthy, fresh, and minimally processed meats when you transition to keto. A study looking at almost half a million people across Europe showed that eating highly processed meats — items like beef jerky and cured meats like deli-style lunch meats — increased the risk of heart disease by 30 percent and also raised the risk of dying from cancer. Unprocessed meats don't carry these risks. The reason for the difference between the two is that processed meats often contain a significant amount of preservatives that can harm the body. Most contain excessive amounts of salt — even for keto dieters who tend to lose salt. Other common preservatives in processed meats include L-carnitine, which may increase the risk of heart disease and heme iron, which is associated with an increase in being diagnosed with diabetes.

Arguably the most important thing to consider when buying a cut of meat is how you're going to prepare it. Most traditional barbeque recipes are out due to the sheer amount of sugar in the sauces, but you may have better luck with dry rubs that emphasize salt over sugar. Instead of focusing on the limitations you have, eagerly explore all the opportunities to try new ways of cooking, frying, smoking, and grilling!

Fishing for fatty seafood

Fish is a great alternate fatty protein source. Most Americans don't get the recommended two servings of seafood per week. On the keto diet, you can buck this trend. Fish is the ultimate source of good-for-you omega-3s and, in addition to being delicious, it's also an excellent source of vitamin D. Many Americans are unknowingly deficient in vitamin D, leading to fatigue, muscle aches, and even a higher risk of bone fractures. Vitamin D is not only vital for bone health, but it also helps improve immune function and may even help with regulating mood. Getting enough fatty fish can significantly increase your vitamin D levels, especially if you live in a colder climate and can't go out in the sun for months at a time. It's best to get wild-caught fish, which often have higher omega-3s and are better for the environment, but farmed fish is still a viable option if you can't afford the expense.

Fatty fish include

>> Salmon

>> Mackerel

>> Anchovies

>> Sardines

>> Catfish

>> Trout

WARNING

Make sure to be aware of mercury, a problematic toxin that can be found in some oily fish like mackerel and tuna. It's more critical for pregnant women and young children to avoid mercury, but everyone should be aware of the potential toxin. Luckily, salmon and catfish are lower in mercury.

Going high-fat in the dairy aisle

Dairy is a good option in keto when you stay away from low-fat options. Never, ever eat low-fat or nonfat dairy, especially those with added fruity flavor, with granola, or sugar-sweetened. Lactose, the primary sugar found in milk, adds to your total carbs, even when you eat non-flavored dairy. Full-fat dairy tends to have a little less lactose than the low-fat variety, but you'll still need to monitor the amount of milk you drink because it can add up quickly.

On the other hand, cheese is an excellent source of keto-friendly dairy, because the liquid whey, which is the source of most of the lactose, is removed. To put it into context, a cup of whole milk has 12.8 grams of carbs, so you really can't have it daily if you want to stay in ketosis, whereas the same amount of cheddar has only 1.7 grams of carbs.

Dairy is also a well-known source of calcium, so you can still enjoy keto-friendly options.

Keto-approved dairy examples include

>> Heavy cream

>> Cheddar cheese

>> Swiss cheese

>> Parmesan cheese

>> Full-fat yogurt (non-sweetened, Greek-style, or cultured)

Hard, aged cheeses tend to have less lactose than softer cheeses. Always default to the hard cheeses on the keto diet. Remember, too, that many commercially available kinds of cheese are filled with artificial ingredients, so choose sharp, aged cheddar (that comes in blocks) rather than the American cheese slices that are only half cheese and mostly processed junk.

When going for butter, you're not restricted to either salted or unsalted. As far as keto is concerned, there are only two things that differentiate between these two options:

>> Whether you're using it for baking

>> Whether you're actively trying to replace your electrolytes

Baking typically calls for unsalted butter so you can control the amount of sodium in your recipe by only using specifically measured amounts. If you need some extra salt (a common occurrence on keto), salted butter may be a better choice. Either way, always try to go for a grass-fed brand; the nutritional quality is exponentially better.

If you get bloating, flatulence, and uncomfortable belly pain with even the smallest amount of dairy, never fear. Keto is perfect if you're lactose intolerant, because you'll need to limit your milk intake, anyway. We cover a number of the best milk replacements in Chapter 6.

Picking the best cooking oils

You'll be sautéing and frying many of your foods on keto, as fat becomes the most crucial macronutrient in your diet. Being aware of the type of oil you use is essential. Most low-quality vegetable oils are filled with inflammatory PUFAs and have been highly processed with chemicals, removing any nutrients that their long-forgotten vegetable predecessors may have had.

On the other hand, minimally processed keto-friendly oils are a must. When you come across high-quality oils, you'll see labels like "virgin," "extra virgin," and "expeller pressed." Here's what these terms mean:

>> **Expeller pressed:** The seed of the vegetable is pressed at high pressures, which can involve high heats.

>> **Virgin and extra virgin:** The oil is mechanically pressed (or more accurately, centrifuged) at lower heats than expeller-pressed methods. Extra-virgin oils are the most expensive because they're "pressed" only once and do not produce a lot of oil. Virgin oils may also be called "cold pressed."

You want to avoid refined oils, which use chemicals and solvents to squeeze out the oils from the seeds cheaply. These oils are the most processed and the least nutritious and tend to be the most common (and cheapest) oils available. You'll often find refined oils in packaged bakery items.

Virgin oils tend to contain higher levels of nutrients, like antioxidants. Virgin oils also have more of the taste and aroma of their parent food, so an extra–virgin olive oil will smell like olives, whereas a refined olive oil will be bland.

The best options are:

>> **Virgin coconut oil:** With more than 90 percent saturated fat, coconut oil is perfect for cooking due to its high smoke point and is unlikely to go rancid, like PUFA-rich oils. What's more, half of its fat comes from medium-chain triglycerides (MCTs), which are a wonderful "fat-burning" fat, meaning it can be a factor in added weight-loss. People who eat high amounts of coconut oil and MCTs also have higher levels of high-density lipoprotein (HDL), which is the "good" cholesterol.

>> **Extra-virgin olive oil:** Derived from the mighty olive, this Mediterranean oil is known for its beneficial MUFAs. People who use olive oil tend to have normal blood pressure, stable weight, and less risk of cardiovascular disease. Additionally, extra-virgin olive oil is known for its high levels of phenols, which are antioxidant powerhouses. The phenols give the oil its characteristic olive-y taste, reduce inflammation, and may be the reason that adding olive oil to your diet can slash your risk of developing several types of cancers. Olive oil is versatile because it has a good smoke point, making it great for frying, and it's also an excellent base for salad dressings and marinades.

>> **Expeller-pressed canola oil:** Although canola oil has gotten some bad reviews, that's mainly because people have been eating low-quality varieties. Refined canola oil — what is often sold in the grocery store — generally has GMOs and is highly processed and even hydrogenated, leading to an increase in artificial (and unhealthy) trans fats. However, expeller-pressed varieties have high levels of good-for-you MUFAs that rival those of olive oil. Also, unlike most other vegetable oils, it has a better ratio of omega-6 to omega-3 fatty acids.

>> **Lard:** Although animal fat like lard often gets a bad rap because of concerns about saturated fat, these concerns are mostly unfounded. In fact, lard has less saturated fat than butter and almost double the amount of healthy MUFAs. Lard is an excellent option for cooking due to its high smoke point.

Avoid eating the lard found on the lowest shelf in your local supermarket. These store-bought options are often highly processed and hydrogenated, increasing the amount of artificial trans fats, which are unhealthy. Instead, search for lard from free-range animals, and specifically, *leaf lard,* which is the least processed fat that surrounds the kidneys and midsection of the animal. Although lard is technically pork fat, other animal fats, such as tallow and duck fat, work just as well.

TIP

Be careful which solid fat you choose. Shortening may contain partially hydrogenated vegetable oils as well as artificial trans fats, so don't choose these to cook or bake with!

An honorable mention is high-oleic sunflower oil. This variety is bred from a seed that has high levels of oleic acid, a type of MUFA that boosts its anti-inflammatory profile. In fact, most varieties have higher MUFA content than olive oil! It also has a high smoke point, making it an excellent option for frying with high heat. Studies show that people who consume these high-oleic varieties show demonstrable improvement in their cholesterol levels. Be aware that both natural and GMO options are available.

Slathering on the butter and mayo

Hold the fat-free mayo and definitely don't eat the margarine. Margarine has a higher association with heart disease than butter, because many varieties still have artificial trans fats. Fat-free mayo is filled with unacceptable thickening starchy agents that will kick you out of ketosis if you aren't careful.

Real mayo is a mix of oil, egg yolks, and vinegar (or lemon juice), so you want to be confident that you get mayonnaise made from one of the best oil sources and eggs from free-range chickens. As a dairy product, make sure you get butter produced from hormone- and antibiotic-free cows. Butter includes all fat-soluble vitamins, including vitamins A and D, which are crucial for eye and bone health.

TIP

An excellent replacement for butter is *ghee*, a clarified (or heated) butter. Ghee has additional benefits — it's high in short- and medium-chain fatty acids and saturated fats that are beneficial for heart health, contribute to increased weight loss, and improve your gut health.

Scoping out other great sources of healthy fats

There are many other great fats on the keto list. The best part is that these alternative fats are whole keto foods because they're either low in carbs or moderate in protein. Avocados, nuts, seeds, and soy-based proteins have other nutrients that will keep you full and expand the flavor, colors, and foods you can eat. For example, did you know that tofu only has 2.3 grams of carbs in half a cup and is a good source of fat and protein? Tofu can be an excellent option for lunch or dinner, or you can use it to thicken keto-friendly smoothies. There are endless options when it comes to fat in keto.

We cover some of these good sources of low-carb proteins in the next section.

Stocking up on healthy proteins

On a moderate-protein diet, you'll have to eat a wide array of animal and vegetable protein sources. Meat, fish, and dairy are a great source of protein and fat, as are nuts and seeds.

In addition to fatty fish, you can also add shellfish to your diet. They contain omega-3s, as well as iron and zinc. Know that some of these protein sources may have more carbs than fish do. Some good low-carb choices are the crustacean group:

>> Shrimp

>> Lobster

>> Crabs

>> Crawfish

>> Prawns

Mollusks tend to have more carbs per serving than crustaceans, so make sure to account for them when you indulge. Like some fish, shellfish can contain mercury, so be sure to find out where your seafood originated and keep your consumption of seafood to about 12 ounces weekly. Here are some popular options in this seafood division:

>> Oysters

>> Mussels

>> Scallops

You'll also want to try some other vegetarian, low-carb options like tofu and tempeh. Both have only about 1 or 2 grams of carbs per serving and have some great benefits. Both tofu and tempeh are made from soybeans and are a complete source of protein because they contain all the essential amino acids. Tempeh is fermented soy (which increases the protein and fiber), while tofu is condensed soymilk that has been mixed with salt-free seawater. Both tempeh and tofu are good sources of minerals like manganese and calcium and are blank slates that absorb the surrounding the flavors, so you can get creative with keto marinades and stir-fries.

Some people are concerned that soy products are unhealthy, but this is generally a misconception. Soy products contain isoflavones, which target the same receptor as estrogen, the hormone critical for female development and reproduction. However, isoflavones are many times weaker than estrogen; they can produce estrogen-like effects or they can have the opposite effect. Studies show that isoflavones are very beneficial — they decrease the risk of cancers like prostate, breast, and colon cancer (the most common three cancers) and are associated with reduced rates of diabetes and heart disease. Be aware, however, that if you suffer from thyroid issues, excess soy may not be a good product for you. Also, it's true that soybeans are often GMO, so if you're concerned about the health benefits of GMO foods, look for organic brands.

Opting for healthier carbs

Not all carbs are created equal. We discuss total carbs and net carbs in depth in Chapter 8, but for now, know that what you need to count is net carbs. When you look at a nutrition label and see "total carbs," you'll also see a line underneath that says "fiber." Because the body can't digest fiber, it passes through without raising your blood sugar. Subtract fiber from total carbs, and what remains will be the carbs you're counting.

Some fruits and vegetables are so high in sugar that they'll never be a building block for keto, but that's okay. There are plenty of other delicious, nutritious, and otherwise appealing options for you to choose from.

Choosing low-carb veggies

Vegetables are necessary for a well-balanced keto diet. As a rule, you'll want to select "above-ground" veggies and stay away from root and tuber vegetables, which are higher in carbs. Low-carb vegetables are a vital source of nutrient-rich vitamins, minerals, and antioxidants on the keto diet. They're invaluable in getting your recommended amount of fiber, so don't skimp on these nutrition powerhouses!

You can enjoy slathering low-carb veggies with keto-friendly dips, sautéing them into a stir-fry, or getting creative and transforming them into keto-friendly "rice" or "noodles."

Some good options include

>> Artichokes

>> Asparagus

>> Leafy greens like spinach, kale, Swiss chard, and arugula

>> Cucumbers

>> Cauliflower

>> Zucchini

>> Broccoli

>> Celery

>> Cabbage

>> Rhubarb

>> Artichokes

>> Onions

>> Garlic

>> Bell peppers

Picking low-glycemic fruits

Low-glycemic carbs are those carbs that are less likely to increase your blood sugar levels and cause an unhealthy rise in insulin. Most fruits are filled with sugar (and fructose), so you have to be careful which fruits you eat, and how much of them. For example, half a cup of blueberries has about 8 grams of carbs, so you'll need to limit any extra carbs on the days you eat these fruits.

Still, there are a variety of fruits you can eat in a modest amount while staying in ketosis:

>> Avocados

>> Limes

>> Lemons

>> Watermelon

>> Honeydew

>> Cantaloupe

>> Berries (blueberries, strawberries, lingonberries, blackberries)

>> Tomatoes

Yes, avocados and tomatoes are fruits. Because their GI is so low, you can load up on these healthy fruits. Besides, both are ripe with nutrients — avocados are rich in fiber and potassium, while tomatoes are known for heart-healthy lycopene.

When choosing your fruits and veggies, it's a good idea to know about the traditional Dirty Dozen and Clean Fifteen — the list by the Environmental Working Group (EWG) that ranks the vegetables that you should always buy organic and the ones that you can buy from conventional farms. The difference is that the

Dirty Dozen is more likely to have pesticides and insecticide residue that won't rinse off with washing or fruit and veggie rinses. You should always buy these foods organic, whereas you can save your money on the Clean Fifteen group.

Because you'll only eat the low-carb and low-GI fruits and veggies, here are the Dirty Six that you should *always* buy organic:

>> Strawberries

>> Spinach

>> Celery

>> Bell peppers

>> Hot peppers

>> Tomatoes

On the other hand, don't waste your money buying these nine in the organic section:

>> Asparagus

>> Avocado

>> Broccoli

>> Cabbage

>> Cantaloupe

>> Cauliflower

>> Eggplant

>> Honeydew

>> Onions

TIP

Spend the extra money for organic keto fruits and veggies in the Dirty Six list.

Squirreling away some seeds and nuts

Nuts and seeds are a perfect keto food — high in fat and a good source of protein. Be aware, however, that the carb content varies and they tend to be higher in omega-6 PUFAs. Nuts are versatile as an on-the-go snack; as an indulgent "breading" for animal proteins; or as "flours" for keto breads, pancakes, and desserts. Nuts you can fill up on (with the number of carbs per ounce serving) are:

- » **Brazil nuts:** 3 grams
- » **Pecans:** 4 grams
- » **Macadamia nuts:** 4 grams
- » **Pine nuts:** 5 grams
- » **Almonds:** 6 grams

Cashews and pistachios tend to have between 8 and 9 grams of carbs per 1-ounce serving, so restrict these options.

A range of seeds is available to add to your keto pantry — flax, chia, hemp, and sesame seeds are all great additions. Like nuts, they can be a great on-the-go snack, as a salad topping, or even as a blend-in for a keto-friendly smoothie. Both nut and seed oils — like walnut oil and sesame oil — can be healthy oils for salads and condiments. Be aware that these oils have higher levels of PUFAs, which have lower smoke points, so they generally shouldn't be used as cooking oil and may need to be refrigerated or stored in a cool, dry cupboard.

Scoping out healthier sweeteners

The keto diet is not known for its sweetness. The upside is that you'll get to indulge in fats and oils. However, once in a while, it's okay to have a little sweet treat, especially as you're transitioning and may still have some cravings for carbs. As time goes on, you'll likely stop craving added sweeteners and be surprised at how sensitive your palate is to the natural sweetness found in whole foods. Until that time, the sweeteners allowed on the keto diet are

- » **Stevia:** A natural sugar-like substitute, stevia is much sweeter than sugar, so a little goes a very long way. It contains no calories or carbs and is available in both powdered and liquid forms. Stevia is very healthy, and studies show that, unlike most other sweeteners, it does not increase insulin levels. Still, it can take some getting used to because it can have a bitter aftertaste. Also, beware of some stevia products that have artificial sweeteners, like maltodextrin, added in.

- » **Xylitol:** A sugar alcohol (like erythritol), xylitol is a complex carbohydrate that the body can't digest well. It's still partially absorbed by the gut, so it isn't entirely carb-free and does cause a smaller insulin spike than sugar. Sugar alcohols are tricky because people react to them differently. Some people can't absorb them well and tend to have more stomach upset — gas and bloating — from the unabsorbed sugar alcohols in the intestine. Xylitol is about as sweet as sugar but with only about half the calories. It's a great option to sweeten your tea and coffee or for baking desserts. Xylitol also has the added benefit of being great for your teeth.

>> **Erythritol:** Another sugar alcohol, erythritol contains only 6 percent the number of calories as sugar, yet is about 80 percent as sweet. It tends to be a bit gritty but it's still a good option for baking. Unlike the other sugar alcohols, however, erythritol does not cause an increase in insulin levels and is also less likely to cause gassiness or bloating.

>> **Monk fruit:** A natural sugar extracted from monk fruit (whose real name is lo han guo), a melon-like fruit found China, it contains no calories and no carbs, yet can be 200 to 500 times as sweet as sugar. Its sweetness comes from mogrosides, which are antioxidant compounds that help decrease inflammation and have antibiotic properties. In fact, monk fruit has been used by the monks who originally cultivated them as a remedy for coughs and other medical complaints for centuries. It doesn't raise blood sugar levels, but its effect on insulin levels is less clear. Some animal studies show an antidiabetic effect while others suggest it may increase insulin levels. The change in insulin levels may be dependent on your sensitivity to insulin, so people who are at risk of diabetes should probably use this sweetener with caution. It can be used to sweeten beverages, as well as in baked goods.

TIP

Some people choose to combine these alternative sweeteners to reproduce the consistency of sugar in baked goods. You may need to experiment a bit, but a common option is combining stevia and erythritol.

Shopping for pre-fab keto products

Pre-fab keto products fall into a couple of different categories:

>> Exogenous ketones

>> Meal prep

>> Meal replacements

>> Supplements

Exogenous ketones

One of the hottest products to hit the keto dieting sphere has been exogenous ketones. *Exogenous* means "produced outside the body"; the ketones your body produces are called *endogenous* (produced inside the body). Exogenous ketones are supplements that promise to flood your body with ketones, getting you into ketosis more quickly the first time; they help you stay in ketosis when you're cutting it close with your carbs, and drop you right back into keto after you've cheated.

The theory is that because being in ketosis produces ketones, proactively flooding your system with them will help you get on the right track faster than waiting for your body to produce them naturally.

This theory makes sense at first, but the more you look into, it the less impressive it becomes. We're huge proponents of basing all our beliefs off of science, and one of the main ways we do that is to take everything back to peer-reviewed studies. This is the standard in the scientific and medical community — when someone has a theory about something, she conducts a study, publishes a paper on it, and then opens it up to the scientific community at large (and her particular field, specifically) for feedback. This is a well-established system that helps ensure multiple independent experts confirm the science we base our lives off of.

Unfortunately, there hasn't been a single peer-reviewed study on the effectiveness of using exogenous ketones for any of these claims. Numerous studies have been run on endogenous ketones (the ones you naturally produce) or on *ketone esters* (a different kind of exogenous ketones; the vast majority on the market are ketone salts, which are very different), but none on the core ketone supplements available.

You may have run into someone in the keto community who swears by exogenous ketones, and it's very likely he has had a positive experience with one; he may tell you about one of the most publicized benefits: increased energy levels. Most of the supplements on the market are packed with caffeine; one popular option we reviewed has as much caffeine as a 16-ounce cup of coffee! Other supplements contain malic acid, known for its ability to increase energy and tolerance to exercise. If the supplement is packed with other ingredients that adequately explain all the benefits you see and feel, it's questionable, at best, whether you're getting any actual benefit from exogenous ketone supplements.

Another thing to consider is diabetic ketoacidosis, which we discuss in Chapter 2. This condition occurs when high levels of insulin (triggered by blood glucose) and high levels of ketones mix in the blood, causing a rapid, dangerous downward spiral in your health. The body is designed to naturally protect against this by not producing ketones until it's the right time.

As you begin the keto diet, you'll eliminate carbs and the body will quickly use up all its glucose stores, then its glycogen stores. After those are gone, your capacity to use glucose for energy is virtually eliminated — because there's no glucose to use, and you're not replenishing your stores. A small amount of glucose is made by the body through gluconeogenesis (covered in Chapter 3), but not enough to trigger a significant insulin release. When the body realizes it's run out of glucose, it signals the liver to begin breaking down fat into ketones and essentially "switch fuels" for energy.

Because blood sugar is eliminated before the body begins making ketones, it's extremely difficult to trigger ketoacidosis in someone who doesn't have type 1 diabetes. However, if someone were to flood her body with ketones before she had eliminated glucose from her system, she would be working against the body's natural processes and potentially entering a dangerous situation.

Finally, remember that the benefit of ketosis isn't having ketones in your system — that's just a byproduct. The primary advantage of ketosis, for most people, is that the ketones are being made (fat is being broken down into ketones, burning up that muffin top you may be struggling with). It's possible to eat too much fat on keto, filling all your caloric needs with what you eat rather than digging into the fat you're trying to burn. In the same way, if you flood your system with exogenous ketones, the body doesn't have a reason to make a tremendous number of these little balls of energy itself, meaning it doesn't burn the fat you're trying to lose.

There are also a significant number of downsides or potential downsides to these supplements. The first is just the sheer expense: The higher-end ketone supplements can cost up to $400 per month for a full regimen. Because the science behind the supplements is either unclear or nonexistent, most companies hide the portions of their ingredients behind tags such as "proprietary blend." The problem with this is that you have no idea how much you're getting in the way of ketones, and that's a significant problem.

Very rarely in life are there effective shortcuts, and this appears to be one of those areas where the slow and steady way still wins the race.

Meal prep

Numerous services offer keto-focused meal prep options; some even give you the ability to customize your macros when you choose your meals. If you live a busy life and just don't have the time or the inclination to cook, these can be lifesavers. One of the temptations of those on the keto diet is to stick to the same few meals and rotate them. In addition to potentially causing food exhaustion, leading to discouragement and a higher chance of abandoning the diet, you can develop nutrient deficiencies in certain areas if you're not consuming a well-balanced diet with a number of different meals. Most meal prep companies that offer keto options use fresh ingredients in all their food, so you're not dealing with anything that's been processed.

Meal prep services provide that variance, even introducing you to dishes you've never tried before. With all their upsides, though, meal prep services do have a few disadvantages, the foremost of which is cost. Ordering meals through a company can cost $8 to $14 per meal, which adds up very quickly. You have to stay on top of the ordering cycle because many prep companies deliver fresh food that's either refrigerated or flash-frozen and requires immediate attention, as well as a resupply every few days or every week. If your company doesn't allow automatic reordering, that's another thing to keep up with — if you forget to put your order in, you may be stuck without any meals and any ingredients with which to make them.

The bottom line is that it's a lifestyle choice. If you're okay with the cost and the scheduling, there's no reason you shouldn't try a meal prep service.

Meal replacements

In this section, we've lumped together every kind of prepackaged keto meal you can get in the frozen foods section of your store. You may be getting a better macros selection, but these frozen meals are often heavily processed and still have all the downsides of regular frozen meals.

Many ingredients are highly processed and contain a number of additives. Because fresh food is such a cornerstone of the keto diet, it isn't great to be filling up with processed items on a regular basis, even if the macros do seem to line up. Speaking of macros, however, we need to discuss what the definition of *keto* is, as far as it's used in the prepared meals section.

There isn't one. That can be a significant problem because *low-carb* could simply mean "lower-carb than our regular options." Sometimes a single "low-carb" meal will have your full daily allotment of carbs; it's technically within your macros for the day and it's lower carb than the standard American diet calls for, but it doesn't mean it's going to help you out very much.

Another problem with processed frozen meals is something called *calorie availability*. Digestion within the body can be divided into two processes: mechanical (your teeth chewing up the food) and chemical (your stomach acids breaking the chewed food down). Fresh ingredients require quite a bit of effort to break apart, and this makes the body work hard for its digestion. Working hard means burning calories, and the harder your digestive system has to work, the more fat you'll burn through.

Processed food tends to be much softer, meaning that it's essentially pre-digested to a large extent. Your body doesn't have to work as hard to break it down, meaning you burn fewer calories. Relying on prepackaged food means that you'll have to decrease your caloric intake to some degree because you'll be retaining more of the calories you consume.

Although food that's within your macros isn't necessarily "bad," there are a substantial number of downsides to relying on frozen or packaged food. Make this the exception, not the rule, and try to cook from fresh ingredients as much as you can.

Several companies have started selling meal replacement shakes that are specifically designed for the keto diet. Think of these as a can of SlimFast (which is one of the companies selling keto shakes); while they shouldn't form the backbone of your diet, they can be useful in a pinch. As long as you stay within your macros and hit your calorie target, there's nothing wrong with occasionally grabbing one of these on the go during a busy week.

The ironic potential downside of these shakes is that it's often difficult to stop at just one or to not eat more food later on because you don't feel satisfied. Although the most important aspect of keto is *what* you're consuming, *how much* of it you're eating also plays a crucial role. Again, you could be firmly in ketosis: Your urine strips show it, your blood tests confirm it, you feel great — but you're not losing an ounce of weight. If you're eating so much that your body has all its fuel needs met from consumed fat, it will never turn to stored fat. Maintaining a caloric deficit (eating a bit less than what your body needs) is still a critical cornerstone of weight loss dieting.

Nutritional supplements

We cover supplements in detail in Chapter 13, but they're worth mentioning here. The first thing you should understand is that supplements exist to *supplement* your diet, not replace it. Ideally, 100 percent of your nutrients will come from your food, and you'll never need to compensate for anything. Realistically, though, this isn't always the case. People have any number of preexisting conditions that could predispose them to various deficiencies, requiring supplementation. Perhaps someone just can't get past the taste of certain foods that are high in a particular vitamin or mineral, eventually leading to a deficiency.

It's important to mention that, because the supplements you choose (if any) should be driven by your body's unmet nutritional needs. Other than a good, daily multivitamin, we don't recommend jumping on any particular supplement proactively. Some vitamins, particularly the fat-soluble ones, can build up in your system over time and lead to problems on their own.

All that being said, there are certain deficiencies that keto dieters are more likely to have than others. The first is a loss of electrolytes: As your body uses up its glucose stores, it loses up to three times the glucose's weight in water. This often carries vital electrolytes out of the body; if you're not actively replacing them, you're going to end up feeling sluggish, uncomfortable, nauseous, and potentially have cramps. Staying hydrated and seasoning your food with salt will go a long way toward resolving this, but it may not address everything. The most common electrolytes to supplement on keto are sodium chloride (salt), potassium, magnesium, calcium, and phosphate.

We cover how the body uses these in Chapter 7, but for this chapter, just know that these are elements you'll need to actively replace when on keto — preferably through your food, but you may need to supplement.

IN THIS CHAPTER

» **Making water your default drink**

» **Loving tea and coffee**

» **Drinking dairy-free milk**

» **Finding flavored beverages**

» **Knowing whether you can drink alcohol**

Chapter **6**

Checking Out Your Beverage Options

I
n this chapter, we cover the best — and worst — drinks on the keto diet, whether you're out on the town or hydrating after an intense workout. Many Americans drink their carbs, in addition to eating them. Sugar-sweetened beverages, whether sodas or sugar-sweetened coffee, will result in unhealthy belly fat and a skyrocketing risk of developing diabetes.

Luckily, keto stops this process in its tracks by encouraging beverages that will leave you toasting to your good health!

Making Water Your Go-To Beverage

Water is an essential part of any nutrition plan. The body is made up of about 60 percent water, so you can't survive without the wet stuff. Unfortunately, too many people aren't getting enough water in their daily lives. Water intake is even more critical on the keto diet because burning fat tends to leave you a little more dehydrated than burning sugar does. As you lose water, salt and electrolytes flow out, so it's vital that you replace these valuable resources throughout the day.

Calculating your water intake

Although you've probably heard the eight-glasses-a-day rule for water intake, the actual amount you need is dependent on a host of factors. Generally, most people should drink between 11 and 16 cups of beverages a day — and the majority of this should be water. If you only drink water (and nothing else), you should be drinking about 9 to 13 cups of water daily.

Generally, men should be at the higher end of this spectrum and women at the lower end of the spectrum. Although there are some physiological differences between the genders, the most significant consideration is body mass. If you're 5'2" and weigh 110 pounds, you'll need far less water than someone who is 6'3" and weighs 240 pounds.

TIP

The best way to remember this is to drink half of your body weight in ounces of water per day. For example, if you weigh 200 pounds, you should drink 100 ounces of water daily. This is only a baseline, though, and your needs may vary.

If you get a cup or two from one of the non-water beverages we cover in the following sections, you can decrease the amount of water you drink. Of course, if you live in a very hot and dry area or you regularly engage in endurance athletics, such as long-distance running, you'll need to drink even more. Also, people living in high altitudes may need to increase their water intake. Generally, if you sweat it out at the gym for an hour, add about another one and a half cups of water to your daily intake.

Flavoring your water with fruits and herbs

Some people balk at the idea of drinking "flavorless" plain water. As kids, drinking water was almost a chore, when there were far more exciting choices, such as chocolate milk and fruit juices, waiting for us in the fridge. Many people still hold onto this nostalgia, thinking that they're wasting their taste buds if they consume plain old water. One of the most common questions we hear is: How can I make myself enjoy water when it's so boring?

Even if you enjoy a cold refreshing glass of ice water, including a little flavor is a great way to spice things up. A slice of lemon or lime is an old standby, but you can add a variety of fruits, like watermelon, berries, or even cucumbers to freshen things up. Cut your favorite fruit into slices or add a handful of berries to a pitcher (or a mason jar to seal in the flavor) and then add water.

INFUSED WATER: HEALTHFUL OR HYPED?

Many contemporary health experts have extolled the virtues of *infused water*, which is water that's had fruit, vegetables, and herbs added to it and soaked for a period of time to extract the flavor. Because it's so popular, it's worth taking a few minutes to dig into these health claims to see what kind of benefits you can realistically expect to experience.

Detox water is infused water that uses recipes supposedly designed to help you remove various toxins from your system. The first thing to understand is that detox water doesn't really detoxify anything: Your kidneys and liver are responsible for filtering toxins out of your body, and they typically do an excellent job of this. Infused water can make it easier for these organs to efficiently filter what you put into your body by maintaining a pH balance similar to what your body naturally maintains.

Blood is typically around a pH of just over 7 (neutral), and the closer you can get to this with your beverages, the less work your body has to do to compensate. Water, of course, has a pH of 7, making it the perfect pairing for maintaining body health. The best thing you can do to detoxify your body is to stay hydrated.

Although detox water isn't a legitimate concept, infused water *does* have some redeeming qualities. The first thing to recognize is that the primary reason for infused water is the second word in the term — getting you to drink more water is the most important benefit of this kind of drink. Infusion simply adds flavor to make it palatable.

Some people claim that infused water can be a nutritional powerhouse, with up to 20 percent of the nutrients from the source fruit leaching into the surrounding water. Even if this were true, slicing up five whole cucumbers to add to your water makes far less sense than, well, just eating one cucumber. Unless you're consuming the food you're infusing your water with, you just don't get many of the benefits those fruits and vegetables offer.

Although many of the benefits of infused water that people claim are fictional, the other thing to consider is that there aren't really any downsides to drinking infused water. If it tastes good, aligns with your macros, and helps you drink more water because of the flavor, go for it! Experiment with different variations until you find the one that is most appealing to your palate.

Did you know you can add herbs to water as well? It's best to add fresh herbs (rather than dry), and cut the herb's leaves to increase the amount of flavor soaking into the water. Great options include rosemary (use sparingly — it's strong!), basil, mint, or thyme.

There are quite a few combinations you can try to wake up your taste buds. Here are just a few:

>> Cucumber, mint, and thyme

>> Watermelon and basil

>> Strawberry and lemon

For all mixes or individual infusions, let the water chill for at least four hours to allow the flavor soak in. These infusions add a little zest to your water, encouraging you to meet your daily requirements, without adding unwanted sugars. Remember to leave the rind on organic citrus fruits for additional flavor.

Adding a no- or low-calorie water enhancer

There are other ways to enhance the flavor of water without using fruit. Remember that the overall goal is to help you drink more water, and as long as you're avoiding anything that will spike your blood sugar or keep you out of ketosis, you've got a pretty wide range of options. Some of these options include

>> **Everly water enhancer:** This is a natural, stevia-sweetened drink mix that is colored with vegetable juice. It comes in caffeine-free and caffeinated options.

>> **Stur Liquid water enhancer:** This flavor enhancer is free of genetically modified organisms (GMOs) and uses stevia for sweetness with a minute amount of fruit or veggie juice for flavor. However, it still manages to remain carb and calorie-free and has 100 percent of your vitamin C requirements. It comes in many flavor options.

Whichever water enhancer you use, make sure to take a look at its ingredient list. It may be no- or low- calorie, but make sure to use a sweetener that is on the keto-approved list. Remember that many of the artificial sweeteners available may end up increasing your blood sugar even if they're technically no-calorie.

Here are a few of the more beneficial (and natural) sweeteners:

>> **Stevia:** This is one of the most popular and well-known natural sweeteners. It's extracted from the leaves of the *Stevia rebaudiana* plant, which is native to South America. Gram for gram, stevia is much sweeter than sugar, so you don't have to use nearly as much of it to achieve the same effects as a much larger quantity of sugar. It has no calories, but it does have several beneficial micronutrients, including chromium, magnesium, potassium, and zinc. Stevia can help to lower blood pressure (as much as 14 percent, according to one

study), and using it as a sugar replacement helps lower blood sugar levels in those with diabetes. Other benefits include lowering low-density lipoprotein (LDL) cholesterol, reducing plaque buildup in arteries, and improving insulin sensitivity. Some people can be sensitive to the taste when it's used in large amounts, but that requires a simple solution: Use less of it!

>> **Erythritol:** This popular sugar alcohol occurs naturally in some fruits and vegetables. It doesn't affect your blood sugar or insulin levels significantly. Because it's a sugar alcohol, erythritol is easy to use as a sugar replacement, especially in baking. It also caramelizes like sugar, so if you have a recipe that calls for this effect, choose erythritol as your sweetener. The downside of this is that, if used excessively, it can cause some digestive issues, so start small and pay attention to the effects it's having on your body.

>> **Monk fruit:** This little fruit is found exclusively in Southeast Asia and has been used by local priests for centuries (hence, the name) as both a sweetener and a medicine. Monk fruit is fascinating because it's the only one in the world that doesn't get its sweetness from fructose; instead, it uses naturally antibacterial substances known as *mogrosides.* Mogrosides pack a powerful punch when it comes to sweetness; at 200 times the sweetness of sugar, a little bit of this goes a long way. Because it doesn't contain any sugar, monk fruit doesn't have any effect on your blood sugar levels.

Less common sweeteners that are still keto-approved include the following:

>> **Yacón syrup:** This sweetener is extracted from the yacón root and, similar to monk fruit, uses something other than fructose for its sweetness. Fructooligosaccharides are the source of this root's sweetness, and they do not raise blood sugar levels.

>> **Chicory root:** This root has been used for centuries and dates back to ancient Rome. Although it's believed to have a number of health benefits, it hasn't been extensively tested.

>> **Tagatose:** This sweetener is commonly found in dairy products; although it isn't zero-calorie, it does contain fewer calories than sugar, but it isn't as sweet.

Those are some of the best sweeteners to use on keto, but here are a few you want to avoid:

>> **Aspartame:** Although this is one of the most commonly used artificial sweeteners, it's also one of the most controversial. Some studies have indicated that it's safe, while other studies have shown a number of adverse side effects, including headaches, dizziness, depression, weight gain, memory

loss, nausea, blurred vision, seizures, and even convulsions. The more severe side effects are only seen in higher concentrations or after a prolonged period of exposure, but the long-term effects of this sweetener remain unclear. When it's used in beverages that are stored in high temperatures, it can quickly break down into the chemical methanol, which isn't great for your body. Because there are better and more natural options available, this sweetener is one we recommend avoiding. If you do decide to use it, avoid cooking or baking with it because of its tendency to break down under high temperatures.

>> **Sucralose:** You may know this sweetener under the brand name of Splenda. It's created by changing the chemical structure of table sugar and is an unbelievable 600 times sweeter than sugar! Sucralose can be an excellent replacement for baking because it retains its sweetness at high temperatures; the downside is that it does contain some carbs and will cause your blood sugar to rise. Unfortunately, very little testing has been done on sucralose to determine its long-term health effects, and some consumers have complained about headaches and thymus gland problems after using it.

WARNING

Although using anything natural is generally preferred to using something that's been processed, there are a few natural sweeteners you should approach with caution. These contain significant amounts of sugar and can negatively impact your ability to stay in keto. Use these sparingly, if at all:

>> Honey

>> Agave syrup/nectar

>> Maple syrup

>> Molasses

>> Dates and date syrup

>> Rice syrup

>> Coconut sugar

Here are a number of sweeteners you should always avoid on keto. Several of these are simply sugar by another name, but we've listed them here so you can have a reference point when you check ingredient lists:

>> Brown sugar

>> Cane juice crystals

>> Cane sugar

- Caramel
- Caster sugar
- Confectioner's sugar
- Corn syrup
- Corn syrup solids
- Demerara sugar
- Dextrose
- Galactose
- Glucose
- High-fructose corn syrup
- Invert sugar
- Muscovado sugar
- Organic raw sugar
- Sucrose
- Turbinado sugar

Sipping on some veggie or meat broth is also an excellent way to include some additional flavor without adding in any unwanted carbs. We've found that this is an excellent choice on a cold winter's morning to keep warm.

TIP

Avoid Crystal Light and other water enhancers that are filled with artificial sweeteners like sucralose. They'll end up raising your insulin levels in the long run.

Adding electrolytes

Keto can increase your water loss, and with it, essential electrolytes like sodium and potassium. Your choice of electrolyte water should include sodium and potassium, as well as magnesium, calcium, and phosphate. Check the label to make sure it provides a range of electrolytes. Peruse the options available at your local supermarket or on Amazon to see which choice has all your needed nutrients.

Here are some good options to try:

- **Liquid sea minerals:** These are concentrated electrolytes from saltwater. Some popular options include electrolytes from the Dead Sea or the Great Salt Lake in the United States. Most have more minerals than you'll know what to do with, but you'll want to focus on the magnesium and potassium because these are the most common deficiencies in the keto diet. Just add a few drops of the sea minerals to your water.

>> **Nuun tablets:** These carb-free tablets provide up to 700 milligrams of sodium for long, high-intensity workouts and also include potassium, calcium, magnesium, and vitamins C and B2 with only about 10 calories and 3 to 4 grams of carbs. Just drop them into your water bottle and rehydrate. They come in a variety of flavors.

Just remember that you shouldn't use these for all your water intake. Even at 3 grams of carbs per serving, if you drink 8 glasses, you likely just consumed all your carbs for the day — and you haven't started eating yet! Use these drinks to supplement your training routine, but select some of the options we mention earlier if you're just looking for additional flavor.

TIP

Adding electrolytes to your water is simple. However you choose to do this, it's a stress-free way to reclaim any minerals and electrolytes by taking them in while focusing on your hydration. It's a no-brainer.

Opting for Coffee or Tea

Coffee and tea are perfectly acceptable choices for keto. Because new coffeehouses or tea places open up regularly, you'll be able to find great options wherever you are. Both drinks are naturally carb-free, meaning you can still enjoy the wide variety of coffee beans and teas while carefully choosing keto-friendly additions to enhance flavor.

REMEMBER

Although coffee and tea are keto-friendly from a carb perspective, they do dehydrate you. If you're managing to stay hydrated, you have a bit more latitude in how much of these delicious beverages you drink. If you're struggling to get your daily water intake in, though, limiting these drinks should be your first step. Staying hydrated is crucial to effective weight loss, and if you're not hitting your goals as fast as you'd like, make sure you're giving your body everything it needs to flush out the waste you produce as you burn through those extra pounds!

Checking out your coffee choices

Coffee is not just many people's go-to beverage to start their day, but it has numerous health benefits, from increasing metabolism and providing a boost of antioxidants to decreasing the risk of colon and lung cancers.

The caffeine found in coffee (and some teas as well) may actually help improve your ability to get into and maintain ketosis. A recent Canadian study that looked at ten healthy adults showed that drinking a cup of joe in the morning increased their production of ketones right away. Caffeine is also known to increase fatty acid breakdown and may play a helpful long-term role in maintaining ketosis.

Coffee, however, is also a diuretic, meaning it increases water (and salt) loss by urination, so make sure you're still keeping up with your overall water intake when you drink coffee.

You've got several options on how to take this dark, tasty beverage:

>> **Black:** Some people love to drink their coffee straight. No calories, no sweeteners, just a shot of caffeine and bold flavor. Numerous studies showing the health benefits of drinking coffee have been published recently. From decreasing your risk of neurodegenerative diseases like Alzheimer's and Parkinson's disease to cutting rates of both liver and colon cancer, coffee can be far healthier than many people realize.

>> **With cream:** Make sure you choose a splash of half-and-half or heavy cream when you indulge in your café au lait. Other dairy products come with excess carbs that can kick you out of ketosis.

>> **With butter, coconut oil, or ghee:** If you're looking for a high-energy breakfast replacement, this is it. Blend well, and enjoy this energy source packed with the mental focus and antioxidants of coffee and the essential nutrients and fats of butter or coconut oil. This can be an excellent option to get you deeper into ketosis because the medium-chain triglycerides (MCTs) from coconut oil and coffee may work together to produce more ketones.

>> **With a zero-calorie sweetener:** This is a good option if you find it hard to drink coffee without a sweetener. You can use one of the keto-approved additives. Over time, as your taste buds develop, you may find you need less sweetener or even none at all.

Considering your tea selections

Like coffee, tea is an antioxidant powerhouse. It has been brewed and drunk for thousands of years with benefits accruing in regular tea drinkers. Most varieties (except herbal) come from the plant *Camellia sinensis*, which is the source of tea's *polyphenols* (plant-based antioxidants that are also found in coffee) — specifically, catechins and epicatechins. Studies show that regular tea drinkers tend to have a low risk of diabetes and heart disease.

There are several types of tea:

>> **Black:** This type of tea is fully oxidized and has the highest levels of caffeine, which can be as high as 80 milligrams per cup, although it generally will be around 50 milligrams, compared to the average of 110 milligrams in coffee. Black tea is a good option if you want a smaller jolt of caffeine to start your day.

>> **Green:** Green tea is not oxidized at all; instead, it's steamed or pan-fried, which leads to higher levels of polyphenols than black tea has (and is why green tea is considered the healthiest). It tends to be more flavorful than other options. Green tea has about a quarter of the amount of caffeine that coffee does.

>> **Herbal:** There are a range of "herbal teas" that may not have any component of *Camellia sinensis,* but tend to have healthy herbs and spices like cinnamon, echinacea, and chamomile, all of which have health benefits — whether you have a cold or you want caffeine-free energy. If you'd like natural sweetness without any added sugar substitutes, seek out these satisfying herbal teas without any extra sugar. Good options are teas that include cinnamon, orange peel, or rooibos varieties. You won't miss the sugar at all.

As with coffee, you can drink your tea:

>> **With cream:** Like coffee, only make a latte with low-lactose varieties of creamer. Never choose the non-dairy powder creamers — they're packed with excess carbs. When prepared correctly, tea lattes are a keto-friendly and decadent way to enjoy your tea on the go.

>> **With a zero-calorie sweetener:** Again, this is an alternative if you have a sweet tooth and don't like plain tea. Make sure to choose only the keto-friendly sweeteners that we discuss in Chapter 5.

Finding a Suitable Milk Replacement

Milk replacements cater to people with lactose intolerance, those who want to avoid dairy for other health reasons (such as hormones and the controversy regarding increased inflammation), or vegans. Because such a wide range of options exist, you should always be able to find one that will leave you satisfied and not missing dairy milk at all.

Make sure always to choose the unsweetened versions of plant-based milks, because sugar-sweetened vanilla and other varieties will rapidly increase your carb intake in no time at all.

Most milk replacements come fortified with calcium to mimic the naturally occurring calcium in dairy milk. Here are your options:

>> **Heavy cream:** It's dense and decadent, and with 38 percent fat, heavy cream is a well-deserved indulgence when you cut out all the sugars of the standard American diet. It's great to add to your coffee, eggs, or rich keto desserts. If you're feeling particularly adventurous, you can even use it to make your own keto-friendly, low-lactose cheese. Remember that heavy cream does come with some associated lactose — up to 8 grams per cup — so use it sparingly in your beverages or cooking.

>> **Almond milk:** This is very popular as a milk alternative. Although almonds themselves are an excellent source of protein, almond milk is primarily water and a small number of pureed almonds, limiting the potential protein intake you can count on from this beverage. Unsweetened varieties generally contain less than 2 grams of carbs per cup, so you can indulge in it. Almond milk is naturally rich in vitamin E and usually fortified with calcium and vitamin D, providing excellent sources of these nutrients as you cut back on dairy milk. Be aware of additives in store-bought brands that often have controversial carrageenan, a thickening additive in many plant-based milks, which may cause gastrointestinal (GI) issues in susceptible people.

Almond milk is very easy to make. Place a cup of raw almonds in a bowl; then fill it with enough water to cover the nuts. Soak for at least 12 hours. When you're ready, drain the water and place the almonds in a blender with 3 cups of fresh water. You'll use the blender in two cycles: For the first cycle, just turn it on low for about ten seconds to break up the nuts. After ten seconds, shut it off to allow the mixture to settle; then blend on high for a full minute. Then strain the mixture through cheesecloth into a bowl. If you want sweet almond milk, return it to the blender and add your favorite no-calorie sugar alternative (monk fruit and/or erythritol work great here!), and then blend until smooth!

>> **Coconut milk:** Coconut milk has the highest fat content of plant-based milks, while still keeping the carbs to 2 grams or less. Coconut is a more decadent milk alternative and, like heavy cream, is a great addition to your cooking and desserts. Like coconut oil, it contains MCTs, which may help with ketosis and weight loss. Be aware that commercial products often contain carrageenan.

>> **Cashew milk:** Like other nut milks, cashew milk is made from the strained pulp of the nut and added to water. It's also low in protein (less than 1 gram per serving) and low in fat (2 grams per serving). This and other nut-based milks are not good options if you have a nut allergy.

» **Flax milk:** Made from cold-pressed flaxseeds, flax milk provides the alpha-linolenic acid (ALA) variety of omega-3 fatty acids (which are not as effective as docosahexaenoic acid [DHA] and eicosapentaenoic acid [EPA]), but like almond milk, flax milk doesn't contain much protein. It's still low in carbs, though, so it's an acceptable option.

» **Hemp milk:** Made from high-protein hemp seeds, hemp milk has a moderate amount of protein for plant-based milk — about 5 grams per cup. It's got more fat as well, at about 7 or 8 grams, and it's very low in carbs. This makes it a closer rival to dairy milk (regarding fat and protein) than the more popular almond milk. It's a good option for those who want a more well-balanced milk alternative. Hemp milk has a slightly nutty flavor and is somewhat creamy, so it does take a bit of getting used to.

» **Soy milk:** Soy milk is a good option for a moderate amount of protein in a plant-based milk. A cup of soy milk has about 7 grams of protein — almost equivalent to dairy milk. It does have a higher carb count than some other plant milks, but this only comes to about 4 grams of carbs per cup. It has the same isoflavones as other soy products, which may provide long-term health benefits. However, it's important to remember that soy is often GMO, so look for a non-GMO soy milk if this concerns you.

Considering Alternatives to Fruit Juice and Soda

Water should be your go-to drink on the keto diet, but you can steer away from this tried-and-true beverage occasionally. Fruit juice and sodas are way too high in sugar to consume on keto, but there are some alternatives you can try to give you a little taste of the sweetness now and then.

REMEMBER

Water should always be the foundation of your fluid intake. To understand why this is so important, you have to wrap your mind around what's going on at the cellular level. When fluid enters your body and begins to interact with your cells, one of three things happens based on what kind of liquid you just drank:

» **The liquid doesn't add water to your system (hydrate you) or take water from your system (dehydrate you).** These kinds of liquids are known as *isotonic;* they have approximately the same salt content as your cells. Sports drinks (such as Gatorade, Powerade, and Vitamin Water) are designed to be isotonic. You should typically only make a habit of drinking isotonic liquids if you find you need to supplement some of the vitamins and minerals they provide, or if you're engaging in strenuous exercise that's making you sweat. In these cases, you're losing nutrients that sports drinks can provide.

>> **The liquid takes water from your system (dehydrates you).** These liquids are known as *hypertonic;* they contain more salt and sugar than your cells have, so they take water from your cells to achieve a balance within your body. Fruit juices and energy drinks are examples of hypertonic liquids. Again, any of these can be fine (as long as they don't exceed your allowable carb intake!), but you need to consume them in moderation to avoid chronic dehydration.

>> **The liquid adds water to your system (hydrates you).** These liquids are known as *hypotonic;* they contain less salt and sugar than your cells have, so they add water to your cells to achieve a balance within your body. Water is the best example of a hypotonic liquid, and it should be your go-to drink. The body needs plenty of fluids to flush waste products. Plus, adequate hydration levels keep your colon moving everything along nicely, helping you to avoid unpleasant, embarrassing, and potentially painful constipation.

Avoiding diet sodas

Just say no to disease-causing diet sodas. They may technically have no calories, research shows that, like their high-carb cousins, diet sodas are just as likely to cause weight gain and long-term health issues. The artificial sweeteners used in diet sodas can stimulate insulin production — even in the absence of glucose — causing the problems of weight gain and insulin resistance even when you don't take in the sugar. Also, diet sodas tend to cause overeating later, whether because your body increases your hunger cues or because you subconsciously justify extra calories because, after all, it was only *diet* soda. Finally, diet sodas often use the worst zero-calorie sweeteners, like aspartame, which is associated with adverse health outcomes, such as headaches and osteoporosis (weak bones). This particular sweetener also isn't entirely off the hook for significant concerns like cancer — it's associated with an increased risk of blood cancers in men.

Shopping for keto-friendly energy drinks

If you're looking for an energy drink that works on the keto diet, give these a try:

>> **Watered-down fruit juice:** This option gives you some of the sweetness without (as many) calories. Still, beware of how many carbs you're getting when you water down the juice; make sure to count them, because they add up more quickly than you may realize. It's probably best to water down juice only around the times you exercise and opt for fruit-infused water at other times.

>> **Powerade Zero:** This drink provides a source of some electrolytes (primarily salt) without the carbs of regular Powerade. It uses sucralose and acesulfame potassium as sweeteners, neither of which raise glucose levels. However, both of these sweeteners can increase insulin levels, making them a bad choice for people who want to lose weight or who are concerned about developing type 2 diabetes. Also, because both are much sweeter than sugar, make sure not to overuse them — your taste buds may become more accustomed to sweetness and leave you craving the sugary taste. Non-sweetened electrolyte drinks may be a better regular option when you exercise. Also, Powerade uses GMO crops, which may be associated with health concerns.

>> **Zero-calorie vitamin water:** The stevia- and erythritol-sweetened version of Coca-Cola's Vitamin Water contains vitamin C and several B vitamins. Although it does contain potassium and calcium, these occur only in trace amounts, but it does provide 25 percent of your zinc RDA. It has about 4 grams of carbs per 20-ounce bottle as well.

>> **Wave Soda Sparkling Juice:** At 6 grams of carbs and just under 50 milligrams of caffeine per 12-ounce can, this low-calorie caffeine kick is a good option for a workout. You shouldn't chug it regularly, but it's a good option if you want some sweetness and you're willing to sacrifice a few carbs for it.

>> **Hint Water:** A convenient fruit-infused water with no sugar or carbs, this is an excellent option if you want to take your fruit water on the go. There are a host of varieties, making it an excellent opportunity to explore exciting taste combinations.

Drinking Alcohol on the Keto Diet

Alcohol and keto can mix — in moderation. Alcohol, like fat, carbs, and protein, is also a source of energy. In fact, alcohol gives you 7 calories per gram, making it more energy dense than both protein and carbs! These are empty carbs, however, and although they can provide a short-lived burst of energy, you're not getting any nutrients, vitamins, or minerals from them. The body doesn't consider alcohol to be an essential macronutrient, so the liver treats this fourth "macro" a bit differently than the others.

Like most things keto, alcohol consumption is about more than just the carb count. Because the ketogenic diet is so firmly rooted in science, the more you understand how your body's biological processes are designed to work, the better off you'll be. There are three main effects you should consider: what alcohol does to your carb count, what it does to your hydration, and what it does to your metabolism.

The easiest factor to calculate is your carb count: You can look at a bottle of your favorite mixer and easily discover how many carbs you'll be consuming with each margarita. These add up quickly, but we've got some great tips to stretch your allowed carbs to their absolute limits.

The second-easiest aspect of alcohol to understand is how it affects your hydration levels. Alcohol dehydrates you, pure and simple. Plan on consuming at least twice the amount of water as the number of alcoholic beverages you'll drink to maintain where you want to be hydration-wise.

Finally, understanding how alcohol affects your weight loss at a biological level is critical. Although alcohol is only toxic in extremely high amounts, the body views it as a toxic macronutrient and will shut down all other digestive processes to metabolize the alcohol and get it out of your system. This is good news to some degree, because metabolizing alcohol is what gives you that "buzzed" feeling. When you're on a high-carb diet, much of the glycogen stores in your body are housed in the liver, where they're being metabolized along with any alcohol you consume. Because so much is going on, you'll metabolize alcohol more slowly and you won't notice the effects as quickly. When you're in ketosis, however, you've cleared out those obstacles and will begin feeling the effects of alcohol much more rapidly.

This isn't good news, however, if you're trying to lose a significant amount of weight and you're used to a regular nightcap. Because the body shuts everything else down to metabolize the alcohol, every 24 hours you're essentially stopping your body's fat-burning abilities, interrupting the process not only at that moment but also preventing yourself from building up any momentum. This can severely slow your weight loss efforts.

Another thing to consider is how alcohol affects your thought processes. We know that alcohol lowers inhibitions and impairs judgment, making the likelihood that you'll cheat on your carbs much higher without being intentional about it. Studies have also shown what will likely come as no surprise to you: When you're intoxicated, you crave high-carb, empty-calorie "filler" foods rather than healthy choices — it's no wonder that Taco Bell and Little Caesars are open after last call, but few salad bars are.

Drinking in moderation is the key. Understanding what each drink "costs" you in terms of carb counts, hydration, and how it affects your metabolism will help you make educated decisions and keep you on the right track to achieving your weight loss goals.

PLANNING AHEAD FOR CRAVINGS

If you're anything like us, you get hungry when you drink. Like all things low-carb, an ounce of preparation goes a long way. Because you know your likelihood of wanting to snack will drastically increase, take a few moments to prepare a few foods you're likely to want when you've had a couple of drinks.

Salty options include the following:

- Hummus with pork rinds, celery, or peppers
- Moon Cheese (puffy, crispy cheese puffs)
- Jerky
- Bacon
- Nuts
- Jalapeño poppers
- Guacamole and pork rinds

Sweet options include the following:

- Chocolate avocado pudding
- Keto lava cake
- Frozen berries
- Chocolate bark
- Keto ice cream

There are plenty of keto-approved possibilities to help ensure you have a fun night without simply deciding to go without. Plan ahead, decide what you're going to eat and drink, and then enjoy yourself!

Leaning toward the low-carb options

A range of alcohols are available that are very low–carb or don't have any carbs at all. These are your best bet to stay in ketosis:

>> **Hard liquors:** These include tequila, rum, vodka, gin, and whiskey, which are all carb-free. Hard liquors are excellent options for the keto dieter on occasion. You can feel free to add low-carb mixers to these, like seltzer water or even Wave Soda.

>> **Dry wines:** Both red and white dry wines contain about 3 to 4 grams of carbs in a typical 5-ounce glass. Luckily, you'll be able to enjoy a toast or two of these keto-friendly options when the occasion arises. Some of the best choices for red wine are Cabernet Sauvignon, Pinot Noir, and Merlot. Pair these with a steak, and you'll be sure to enjoy your night out! Approved white wines include Pinot Grigio, Sauvignon Blanc, Chardonnay, Riesling, and Champagne.

>> **Light beers:** These are generally around 3 grams of carbs per 12-ounce bottle or can as well. They're light on carbs and flavor, which is great if you want a mild taste. Although light beers were first introduced to the market decades ago (and trust us, the first attempts were truly horrible), brewers have made incredible strides in preserving taste and full-bodied integrity. Some of the more popular options we've found include Bud Select 55, Bud Select, MGD, Rolling Rock Green Light, Michelob Ultra, Miller Lite, Natural Light, Michelob Ultra Amber, Coors Light, Amstel Light, and Bud Light.

Avoiding the high-carb options

People often forget the amount of sugar that many mixed drinks have, which can quickly destroy an otherwise keto–friendly lifestyle. Don't let a night out ruin an excellent start to your keto journey.

Drinks that include soda, juice, or other sugars, including the following, should be avoided:

>> Sweet wines, such as Moscato, port, sherry, dessert wines, sangria, and Zinfandel

>> Sugary mixers, like triple sec, whiskey sour mix, blue curacao, grenadine, margarita mixes, and simple syrup

>> Flavored alcohols, including coconut rum, peach or peppermint schnapps, and Baileys Irish Cream

>> Juices, such as cranberry, orange, pineapple, tomato, apple, clamato, blueberry, and grapefruit

>> Energy drinks, such as Red Bull

>> Sodas, which can raise your glycemic index even if you're choosing a low-calorie diet option

>> Liqueurs, such as amaretto, Kahlúa, sambuca, Campari, Cointreau, and Frangelico

>> Fruit add-ins, including cherries, orange slices, pineapple wedges, and various berries

>> Wine coolers

>> Regular beers

Choosing a chaser

Few people are hardcore enough to enjoy straight alcohol, so in addition to the mixers listed earlier, it isn't uncommon to use a chaser. Many of the more popular chasers, such as soda or beer, have a high amount of carbohydrates.

Some keto-approved options are

>> Seltzer water

>> Flavored seltzer water

>> Diet tonic water

>> Diet flavored bubbly water

>> Stevia or erythritol (if you're drinking at home — you'll get a weird look if you ask a bartender for these)

>> Zero-sugar drinks, such as Red Bull Sugar-Free, Bai5 sweetened with erythritol, diet sodas, and sugar-free Monsters

>> Stur (but avoid the ones with aspartame)

>> Mio Water Enhancement

DEALING WITH THE AFTERMATH

Depending on how much you've had to drink, the morning after could be a non-event or a significant roadblock. Coping with a hangover and staying in ketosis is relatively straightforward: Drink more water. When you're done with that, drink some more water. After you've knocked that out and want a change of pace for your day, well, drink more water.

Taking aspirin won't hurt you at all, so if it feels like there's an army of dwarves hammering inside your skull, don't hesitate to pop a few. In the meantime, however, continue drinking water!

Remember: You don't have to give up alcohol to go keto. The two can mix if you're smart about it. Make sure to be smart about which drinks you choose so it doesn't cause undue damage to your keto journey.

IN THIS CHAPTER

» **Getting on track with your keto targets**

» **Sticking to your macro goals**

» **Prepping meals**

» **Snacking smart**

» **Staying hydrated**

Chapter **7**

Achieving Ketosis Step by Step

I n this chapter, we walk you through defining your keto goals one step at a time. Here, you take steps toward clarifying your personal intentions for keto, as well as planning a road map to reach your objectives. A common reason people are unable to achieve their goals is a lack of planning. You may be very excited to jump headfirst into keto, but it's crucial that you begin the journey with a clear plan so that you don't lose steam — and your way — as the weeks progress.

Another important part of sticking to keto is making sure that you don't get into a rut in the kitchen. When a person first transitions into low-carb living, it's common to stick to eating the same two or three items day in and day out. When you approach keto this way, you can easily get bored and feel like you're missing out on numerous tasty options. In this chapter, we include tips to help you stay satisfied while sticking to your calorie and macro limits, as well as explain how to make the lifestyle work day to day by preparing and eating meals that will get and keep you in ketogenic bliss.

If you enjoy snacking, you'll love the tasty and easy-to-prepare options we offer for on-the-go eating that won't use up all your carb allotments. Whether you enjoy salty, sweet, or a little savory, keto offers a number of delicious options.

Personalizing Your Keto Goals

Before cleaning out your pantry or stocking up on avocados and coconut oil, you need to ask yourself the single most important question of your keto journey: "What do I hope to gain from going keto?"

Everyone's answer will be slightly different, and you need to determine your unique reasons for pursuing such a vital lifestyle change. If you view keto as just another diet to try or you choose it because it seems to be a fun trend, it'll be that much harder to commit to the lifestyle. In Chapter 1, we mention a few of the obstacles that you may encounter with keto — and we go over them in detail in Part 3. You'll be much more likely to overcome these challenges if you have a good reason for starting keto in the first place. We firmly believe that you need to be committed if you plan to pursue keto over the long term.

Ask yourself if any of these scenarios fit with your desire to pursue keto:

>> Do you want to lose weight that you haven't been able to shed no matter how much you exercise or diet?

>> Have you tried other diets with no success?

>> Do you struggle to build muscle or tone up even if you really don't have any weight to lose?

>> Do you want to treat a condition you already have, like high cholesterol?

>> Are you eager to prevent future illnesses that you're at risk for, like diabetes or obesity?

TIP

Take a few moments to get very clear on your goals for keto. We found it really helpful to write down our personal hopes for entering this diet. It makes it simple to take stock of where you are in your journey as time goes by. Plus, it helps you recommit to the "why" during difficult parts of transitioning to keto.

Whatever your reason for going keto, it's likely that this lifestyle change can help you achieve your goals. Let's dive in and see how keto can fit into your specific lifestyle and get you where you want to be.

Setting your weight goals

Close your eyes and imagine stepping out on a bright summer day with your jeans perfectly fitted and the confidence of knowing that you not only look good, but also feel amazing. Ask yourself the following questions:

>> Do you have a dream weight (or range) that you've been trying to achieve for a while?

>> Is it realistic?

>> What's your weight now, and how far away are you currently from this dream goal?

>> What's your ideal timeline for achieving your goal weight?

If your goal is in a healthy range, and one in which your body will naturally thrive, keto can help you achieve that vision. A quick way to check this is to determine your ideal body mass index (BMI), which looks at your weight and height to define a normal range of body weight for you. Normal BMI can include a wide range — often more than 30 pounds — so you need to find the weight at which you feel your most energetic and healthy. BMI isn't perfect (your BMI might be in the "overweight" range if you're just extremely muscular, for example), but it's still a handy tool.

TIP

Head to www.nhlbi.nih.gov/health/educational/lose_wt/BMI/bmicalc.htm to calculate your weight. The website also has BMI tables (www.nhlbi.nih.gov/health/educational/lose_wt/BMI/bmi_tbl.htm), which can help you figure out if your dream weight fits into a healthy range for your body.

Ketosis puts you into a state where your body will use the food you eat, as well as extra body fat stores, for energy; along the way, you'll reach your ideal body weight. As we discuss in Chapter 3, ketosis causes your body to become a fat-burning machine. So, instead of storing unhealthy belly fat, you'll burn fat for fuel, creating a leaner and more sculpted you. Keto also helps you lose weight faster than traditional low-fat diets, helping you to stay motivated to stick to your healthy changes. The bonus: You get to lose weight while eating fatty, decadent foods that keep you satisfied!

A lesser-known fact is that keto is also a valid option to maintain or even gain healthy weight. Because ketosis helps you get to your ideal weight, if you're underweight, you'll be able to put on much-needed pounds. If you don't have any weight to lose, make sure you're not cutting calories on keto. Whatever diet you choose, if you drop calories too drastically or in an unsafe way, you run the risk of experiencing adverse outcomes such as hair loss, unhealthy skin, and damage to your liver, kidney, and other organs.

If you want to bulk up, you may choose the targeted ketogenic diet to help gain extra muscle. You can gain weight on the standard ketogenic diet (see Chapter 1), but most studies show that you're unlikely to build — although you can maintain — muscle on the standard version of the diet.

TIP

Whichever type of keto diet you choose, the important point is to focus on high-quality nutrients in all your meals. This is easy to do on keto, because your extra calories will be coming from whole foods that pack a powerful nutritional punch. Adding extra avocado slices, drizzling olive oil on your food, or crunching a handful of walnuts over your lunch salad will give you the calories you need to reach your ideal weight. Its benefits don't stop there, though: Sticking with a diet filled with healthy fats will also add antioxidants, vitamins, and minerals that will leave your hair, skin, and nails glowing while providing nutrition to your brain, liver, and other organs.

REMEMBER

Whatever your weight goals, you'll need to take time to add exercise into your regular routine. Exercise — in addition to a well-balanced keto lifestyle — will ensure that you reach your goals. Not only does exercise improve your heart health, boost your mood with powerful endorphins, and help you sleep like a baby, but it's also critical in helping to shape and tone your body. If you're looking to lose weight, high-intensity cardio and resistance training are vital to dropping extra pounds. On the other hand, if you want to pack on extra muscle, you should consider incorporating more resistance training and increasing the time you spend lifting heavy weights.

Another important concept you'll want to consider is how often you eat. We made the choice to do a mini-fast at the beginning of our keto journey, and that really can help to kickstart your journey by using up all your body's glucose stores and priming you for quick fat burning. Intermittent fasting (which we dive into in Chapter 12) is also an excellent option for helping you speed up your weight loss on the keto diet and has a number of health benefits to boot.

Most people think of intermittent fasting as a tool to help you lose weight, but if you're smart about your options, you can intermittently fast and still gain muscle, because there are many ways to fast. If fasting isn't for you, eating more frequently — whether in a specific eating window or throughout the day — can help you increase your weight gains as well.

This is the time to get clear on your goals and think realistically about how — or if — you want to change your weight when you begin keto. Don't get too caught up on a specific deadline to achieve your weight goals. It's crucial to remember that keto is a lifestyle, not a trendy diet, and its best to go in with a long-term view for your weight journey.

Still, it's best to calculate the number of calories you'll need to eat to reach your weight goals and compare that honestly with how many calories you currently eat. Figuring out the difference between the two will help you develop a plan of attack to make the numbers align in a way that works for you. Incorporating exercise and possibly fasting will help you achieve these goals in a more dynamic fashion that fits your lifestyle.

When you get into the swing of keto, you'll likely find that your body naturally moves toward a healthy weight without too much effort.

TIP

Keto is an excellent tool to help you reach your healthy dream weight. You'll need to get clear on how much weight you want to gain or lose and come up with a realistic plan that looks at your calories, macros, exercise level, and meal frequency to get you to your goal.

Targeting specific health conditions

Keto provides a range of health benefits, any of which is a great motivation for choosing a keto lifestyle. The most common reason people prefer keto — apart from optimizing their weight — is for its benefits with blood sugar control. If you have type 2 diabetes or prediabetes and you've been told to "watch your sugars," keto is an excellent choice to get your blood sugar back to normal levels.

Type 2 diabetes happens because the body has been exposed to high glucose and insulin levels for so long that insulin stops doing its job. This condition is known as *insulin resistance* or *insulin insensitivity.* In this case, blood sugar continues to rise even when insulin levels are high. More than 20 million Americans have been diagnosed with type 2 diabetes, and many millions more have the condition but just don't know it yet. This disease used to be called "adult onset diabetes," but things have changed: Hundreds of thousands of children have developed the disease, mostly brought on by eating sugary snacks and tons of carbs.

Many nutritionists and doctors are seeing the benefits of a keto lifestyle in people with type 2 diabetes. The old recommendations for low-fat, high-carb foods haven't been able to reverse the disease. Many people with diabetes have been able to reduce or even eliminate all their medications and have normal blood sugar after committing to keto.

WARNING

If you already take blood-sugar-lowering medication, talk with your doctor before going low carb because the keto diet works *so* well that diabetes medication can cause an unsafe drop in your blood sugar level.

In Chapter 2, we mention the many other diseases that keto can help to treat:

>> Abnormal cholesterol levels

>> Insomnia and other sleep issues

>> Acne

>> Polycystic ovarian syndrome

>> Migraines and/or cluster headaches

>> Fibromyalgia

>> Seizures

>> Neurodegenerative diseases like Alzheimer's and Parkinson's

If you're tired of being tired, or you're sick of food cravings, brain fog, and generally feeling poorly, keto can overcome this drudgery by providing more energy, freedom from cravings, and mental clarity. Keto is also beneficial for people suffering from chronic inflammation, whether it shows up as acne scars, chronic pain, or even cardiovascular disease. By harnessing the whole-food, anti-inflammatory properties of keto, you're setting yourself up for a lifetime of health that will keep many of the most common causes of death and disease in the United States from taking a toll on you. Keto should always be a choice if you have a health challenge you want to overcome.

WARNING

That said, if you have a major medical condition or you have one of the following problems, it's best to chat with your doctor before pursuing keto. If any of the following conditions apply to you, you may ultimately be able to thrive on the ketogenic diet, but be cautious before jumping in:

>> **Pregnancy or breastfeeding:** Some women follow the keto lifestyle during pregnancy, but it's probably not best to begin your transition onto keto during this time. Pregnancy leads to a host of changes in a woman's body, and adding an extra variable to the mix may lead to unintended consequences for both mother and baby.

Most studies on keto have been on animals — and are, therefore, not directly relatable to humans — but the results have been mixed, with some studies indicating phenomenal health for both mother and baby, and excellent growth rates for the child; other studies have suggested that ketones can negatively impact fetal development.

Also, pregnancy and breastfeeding are two of the rare times that ketoacidosis can occur in a person without diabetes. Researchers think this can happen because the mother's body is so metabolically active caring for the baby that ketosis can get much closer to starvation, triggering ketoacidosis.

>> **Kidney disease:** This one is a bit controversial. Newer research clearly shows that kidney disease, a common long-term complication for people with diabetes, can be delayed by the keto diet. However, other studies show that keto can cause an increase in painful kidney stones, which can worsen kidney function. The increase is likely related to the dehydration commonly associated with ketosis, as well as a relative increase in protein load. Both issues may be harder to combat if you have kidneys that are poorly functioning to begin with. If you have a history of kidney stones, you'll want to be extra

cautious if you experience back or belly pain that suggests an impending stone and increase your fluid (and lemon) intake.

Beware of anyone who says that the keto diet is a poor choice for kidney health because it's high in protein. This is a misconception and has no bearing on people who eat moderate levels of proteins on their keto journey — which is what keto is supposed to be. People with kidney disease shouldn't eat too much protein because this increases the workload of the kidneys. Of course, this does mean that you shouldn't choose the high-protein version of the keto diet if you have kidney problems; studies have shown damage to the poorly functioning kidneys when protein intake is higher than 35 percent of caloric intake.

>> **Liver disease:** This is another controversial area, with studies showing varying results. The liver is the powerhouse of the keto diet because it processes the fats you eat and helps to produce the ketones your body runs on.

Some studies show that the keto diet may cause too much stress on the liver and can lead to the accumulation of fatty deposits and signs of inflammation in the liver. This condition is called non-alcoholic fatty liver disease (NAFLD), and it's one of the most common causes of long-term liver problems. However, other research shows that NAFLD, which tends to be more common in people who rely too heavily on high-carb foods, can actually be treated by choosing a keto diet because it removes the problem: carbohydrates.

NAFLD is sometimes thought of as the liver's version of insulin resistance, so it does make sense that a ketogenic diet — which combats this issue — would help to improve NAFLD. Several studies have indicated that sticking to keto if you have this form of liver disease for six months or more can potentially reverse the issue. Needless to say, because the jury is still out on this one, it's best to be cautious here.

>> **Pancreatic disease (including type 1 diabetes):** Type 2 diabetes is a poster child for the keto diet, but people with type 1 diabetes should be a little more cautious. If you have type 1 diabetes, or any pancreatic disease that impacts your body's ability to produce insulin, sticking to a keto diet could make your blood sugar drop to an unsafe level, leading to ketoacidosis and other problems.

There are also rare cases of a ketogenic diet triggering severe inflammation of the pancreas. This is more likely to happen if you have certain genetic diseases; although these conditions are rare, some people are asymptomatic so they may not know they have the disease.

It's definitely best to touch base with your doctor if you have a family or personal history of pancreatic disease, especially pancreatitis. Also, because a high-fat diet can help you pass gallstones if you already have them (which we cover a bit more in Chapter 10), and gallstones can sometimes lead to pancreatitis, you should also be cautious if you have a history of gallstones.

As an aside, if you're using keto to treat other serious medical conditions, like epilepsy or certain forms of cancer, you should do so under the direction of your doctor. Keto can lead to shifts in your metabolism that may affect your condition.

Preventing future health problems

If you're healthy with no medical issues, awesome! Now, if you want to stay that way for the next 5, 10, 15 years, or longer, a whole-foods keto diet is a great idea. This is especially true if a lot of your family members have many of the medical problems we discuss in Chapter 2, like diabetes, high blood pressure, or heart disease.

Because keto will maintain your blood sugar at normal levels, decrease daily inflammation, and prevent heart disease, there's no reason not to start keto to prevent future ailments. It's important to have your long-term goals in mind, and starting keto with this much foresight will encourage you to maintain the lifestyle, even if you're at your goal weight or you don't have any health problems that you can see right now.

TIP

Keto is a great choice to prevent future health problems. It's never too early to take active steps to change your health for the better.

Calculating Your Macro Targets

As you start your keto journey, it's a good idea to get a sense of not only how many calories you should consume, but also how much of each macro — fat, protein, and carbs — you should eat throughout the day. Many people are awful at estimating the portion size or number of calories in a typical meal. Portion sizes have increased dramatically over the past few decades, with bagels getting twice as big and a standard "cup" of soda more than tripling in size! The recent decision to label calorie servings in restaurants may help this trend, but all too often this information is hidden away from consumers — to decrease the chance that they'll make the better decision to skip the tub of popcorn with the movie.

If you grossly underestimate the number of calories — and carbs — you're eating, you'll keep wondering why you're having a hard time losing extra weight. Being informed and learning how to accurately estimate the number of calories in your go-to meals, as well as the "innocent" snacks that you may sometimes forget to count, will really help you gain a handle on your target food intake.

After you've got a good sense of how many calories you're *actually* eating, it's time to check out some of the calculators available on the web (see the Chapter 23) to figure out how many you *should* be eating.

If you're eager to figure this out now, we've provided you with the tools to help you "guestimate" these values on a daily basis and walk you through how to do this step by step.

Total calories

Your total daily calories, or resting caloric intake, is the number of calories your body needs each day. This number is also called *resting metabolic rate* (RMR), and it's essentially the amount of energy you need every day to carry out the essential functions of life — building up and breaking down the tissues of your body, breathing, and resting quietly.

Your RMR depends on a host of factors, including weight, lean body mass, age, activity level, gender, and more.

If you've wondered why a friend can eat whatever she wants and never gain an ounce, it could be that she's naturally blessed with a faster metabolism from her parents, or it could be related to an overactive thyroid gland. The thyroid produces *thyroxin*, which is the hormone that most tightly influences metabolic rate. Too much of it can lead to weight loss, while *hypothyroidism* — a more common issue — can lead to weight gain.

On the other hand, if someone gains weight by merely glancing at a cookie, it could be due to one of several reasons. He may be shorter (taller people tend to have higher caloric needs), already overweight (fat is less metabolically active than muscle), or spend his days in a climate-controlled environment (exposure to both cold and heat can jump-start RMR because your body has to do the work to regulate your body temperature, rather than the thermostat).

What you eat also affects your metabolism. Eating and digesting your food requires energy and creates heat. The opposite, starvation diets, actually slow your metabolism down as your body tries to conserve what energy you have. You can drop your metabolism by as much as 30 percent if you slash your calories too quickly, making it difficult to lose the extra pounds you're trying to shed. Interestingly, as we mention in Part 1, by optimizing your body's hormonal balance, keto may derail this tendency to hold onto excess weight even as you cut back on calories.

There are two main ways to determine your RMR:

>> **Indirect calorimetry:** This is the most accurate way to assess your RMR, but it's also more cumbersome and expensive. It's a useful tool if you want the most effective and unique nutritional plan to help you achieve your dream weight.

Indirect calorimetry measures the amount of heat you produce by determining how much gas (carbon dioxide and nitrogen) you exhale. Because these gases are the end products of the majority of metabolism, it gives a very accurate measurement of how much energy you use in a given period.

There are several methods to measure your exhaled gases, but they all require purchasing expensive equipment or setting up an appointment with a personal trainer, nutritionist, or doctor. A commonly used device, BodyGem, is a handheld machine that requires about ten minutes to determine your RMR accurately. Older indirect calorimeters required face masks or lying quietly in a closed chamber in a laboratory. Obtaining this result will run you about $50 to $75.

>> **RMR calculators:** These calculators use complicated formulas that take into account several criteria to come up with a unique number of calories you should consume per day. There are several calculators available to estimate your basal calorie intake, but the accuracy of these calculators can vary by as much as 400 calories per day — almost enough to cause a weight change of a pound per week! The various RMR calculators are more likely to cause a higher degree of inaccuracy in people who are overweight. This happens because most of the formulas use your current weight as a significant part of the calculation. Excess body weight is often fat, which is less metabolically active than muscle and will, therefore, overestimate how many calories you actually need if you're overweight.

RMR calculators aren't as precise as indirect calorimetry, so if you really want an accurate result or you're overweight and serious about weight loss, it might be useful to get the indirect calorimetry done for the best results.

TECHNICAL STUFF

If you're okay with a tiny amount of guesswork, the tried-and-true RMR calculator that many dietitians and nutritionists have used for years is the Mifflin–St. Jeor formula. It's the most accurate calculator with a difference from indirect calorimetry of only about 20 calories per day for a person with a healthy body weight. Similar to other calculators, this number rises in an overweight individual and can be as much as a 150-calorie difference.

Beware that both indirect calorimeters and RMR calorimeters only provide you with the minimal number of calories you need, and they don't account for more activity than would happen if you were lying in bed all day binge-watching Netflix. Physical activity is the best thing you can do to increase your daily caloric intake, and you'll need to remember to modify your total caloric intake based on how much activity you do in a given day.

After you've calculated your RMR, you'll need to figure out your *total daily energy expenditure* (TDEE). This number takes into account the amount of activity you do. Use one of the following numbers, depending on your level of daily activity:

>> **1.2:** You have an office job and spend very little time engaging in any physical activity.

>> **1.375:** You're slightly more active. This generally means doing some walking or household work up to three days a week.

>> **1.55:** You engage in moderate levels of activity. People in this category exercise at a higher level between three and five days a week.

>> **1.725:** You're very active. You enjoy significant exercise, like CrossFit, swimming, or some form of martial arts, six or seven days each week.

>> **1.9:** You're close to an Olympic-level athlete. You can use this number if you have a very physically demanding day job, or you engage in professional-level sports regularly.

If you're trying to lose or gain weight, of course, you need to adjust these numbers to reflect your goal. As a general rule, although there is some variety to these results, you need to slash (or add) about 250 calories per day to lose (or gain) half a pound per week. Bump this up to 500 calories a day if you'd like to move the scale about one pound in a week. The basic math for weight loss takes your RMR, adds in the amount of physical activity you do, and then matches those needs with what you eat. If you have an excess, you'll gain weight; if you have a deficit, you're primed to lose weight.

TIP

Here is the basic Mifflin–St. Jeor formula. It's different depending on your gender:

>> **For men:** (10 × weight in kilograms) + (6.25 × height in centimeters) – (5 × age in years) + 5

>> **For women:** (10 × weight in kilograms) + (6.25 × height in centimeters) – (5 × age in years) – 161

TIP

To convert pounds to kilograms, divide your weight in pounds by 2.2. To convert inches to centimeters, multiply your height in inches by 2.54.

Let's take the example of a man who is 30 years old, weighs 150 pounds, and is 5 feet 8 inches tall. Assume he wants to maintain his weight and he's working a desk job with little physical activity. Here's how to calculate his total caloric intake:

1. **Convert his weight (150 pounds) to kilograms.**

   That's 150 ÷ 2.2 = 68.18 kilograms.

2. **Convert his height (5 feet 8 inches) to centimeters.**

   First, you have to convert his height to inches. There are 12 inches in 1 foot, so he's 60 inches + 8 inches = 68 inches tall. Now 68 × 2.54 = 172.72 centimeters.

3. **Multiply his weight in kilograms by 10.**

   That's 68.18 × 10 = 681.8.

4. **Multiply his height in centimeters by 6.25.**

   That's 172.72 × 6.25 = 1,079.5.

5. **Multiply his age in years by 5.**

   That's 30 × 5 = 150.

6. **Add the amounts from Step 3 and Step 4, subtract the amount from Step 5, and add 5.**

   That's 681.8 + 1,079.5 – 150 + 5 = 1,616.3 calories. That's his RMR.

7. **To get his TDEE, multiply his RMR by 1.2, which reflects his activity level.**

   That's 1616.3 × 1.2 = 1,939.56, or rounding up, 1,940 calories per day.

TIP

If the idea of doing all this math sounds like torture to you, you can find a free online calculator at http://fitcal.me/tdee.

Fat grams

After figuring out the number of calories you need, it's time to take a look at how many grams of each type of macro you should be eating per day. To figure this out, you'll need to multiply your total calories by the fraction the macro plays in your daily diet. For example, if you're consuming 2,000 calories per day and you want to go with 75 percent from fat, 20 percent from protein, and 5 percent from carbs, you'd perform the following calculations:

>> 2,000 × 0.75 = 1,500 calories from fat per day

>> 2,000 × 0.20 = 400 calories from protein per day

>> 2,000 × 0.05 = 100 calories from carbs per day

Unfortunately, most nutrition labels don't break down your macros into calories from each group; they give you the total number of calories, and then break each individual nutrient into grams. That means the next step is finding out how many grams of each macro you can have.

REMEMBER

Your percentage of fat and protein will slightly change if you're on the standard ketogenic diet versus the protein ketogenic diet. Both protein and carbs provide four calories per gram, while fat contains nine calories, so divide by the appropriate number to get accurate results.

As the majority of your caloric intake, fat should be about 75 percent of your total intake on keto. Some people may go as high as 80 percent (strict keto for medical conditions like epilepsy) or drop down to 65 percent (if they're on the high-protein keto diet). Let's continue using the example above:

   1,500 ÷ 9 = 167 grams

In this example, you need to eat about 167 grams of fat per day. You'll need to adjust this depending on the type of keto diet you're following. You divide by nine because there are nine calories for every fat gram, compared to four each for the other two macros.

Protein grams

To calculate calories for moderate protein (for maintenance and weight loss, not building muscle) intake, the formula looks like this:

   200 ÷ 4 = 100 grams

This example, for the standard ketogenic diet, will require about 100 grams of protein. If you're trying to build muscle, the general rule is to take in 1 gram of protein per pound of body weight, although this would decrease if you're significantly overweight.

TIP

If your body fat percentage is 30 percent or higher for women or 25 percent or higher for men, you should focus on losing excess fat before really attempting to build muscle. This isn't to say that you can't go to the gym before you hit a certain body fat percentage — not at all! However, bulking and building muscle requires excess protein, which means upping your overall caloric intake while decreasing the amount of fat you're eating. It can get very complicated to try to balance having enough excess calories to build muscle while cutting them to lose fat. You *can* successfully combine these two efforts, but it's somewhat difficult. If you're just starting out, focus on either fat loss *or* muscle building.

Carb grams

The macro with the least amount of calories will be carbs, and it's calculated by the following formula (again, using the example from earlier):

100 ÷ 4 = 25 grams

Generally, eating around 25 grams of carbs is a good starting point when you decide to transition to the keto diet. However, everyone will have a slightly different carb allotment. Some people will maintain ketosis at a little over 50 grams of carbs per day while others have to really slash their carbs to stay in ketosis. Over time, as you understand when your body is in ketosis (or with the aid of urine strips or other tests), you may be able to modify your carb allotment. Also, if you're on the targeted keto diet and you add some extra carbs around the time of your intense workout, you'll be able to increase this number. Remember that the longer you're on keto, the more efficiently your body uses the process, and you can generally add in more carbs over time.

TIP

A critical part of success on the keto diet is being aware of how many calories you need each day, as well as where you need to get your calories. Pull out your dusty calculator or head over to a good calorie counter to keep yourself on track.

Planning and Preparing Meals

On the keto diet, like any other meal plan, planning is the key to success. You'll want some variety occasionally, but we know all too well how life can get hectic pretty quickly. You may not have an hour, or even five minutes, to make the perfect meal. Unless you have a personal chef, who can whip up keto delicacies on demand, its best to have a plan. We give you some great recipes in this book, but you should have a good sense of what proportion of macros should be on your plate at any given meal.

Generally, having a 3- or 4-ounce serving of a protein source like meat, chicken, or fish (about 20 to 30 grams of protein) is a good start, as well as a choice or two of fat and a heaping of low-carb veggies. This combination can change slightly depending on the meal, your taste preferences, and what your last meal looked like. You may skip the protein or carbs for a snack or one of your meals, but you'll need to keep the fat constant. Because fat is pretty dense (nine calories per gram compared to four each for protein and carbs), you won't always have a larger volume of fat on your plate.

Here are some great examples of keto meals:

>> Greek yogurt and nut butter

>> Egg frittata with mixed veggies, protein, and heavy cream

>> Meat entrée with cream sauce and sautéed veggies

>> Huge salad of greens with nuts/seeds, a meat or veggie protein source, oil-based vinaigrette, and avocado

>> Cauliflower rice with a protein source

Meal prepping is an excellent option for keto. You'll need to set aside an hour or two on a day you have extra time to prepare, and portion your protein, fats, and veggies. It's straightforward just to grab these on the go or make a simple dinner out of your prepped meals in the middle of the week. Many of the recipes in Part 5 can be made on a large scale and saved in the fridge or freezer for the week to help with meal prep. If there is a recipe you genuinely enjoy, this is a great way to get it made and easily within reach a couple of times a week.

This is also the time to get a working knowledge of spices in your pantry. Whether you take a cooking class, search online, or use our recipe section, you'll want to have an array of spices that can up the ante on your proteins and veggies. Understanding how to make a simple vinaigrette or marinade is essential to creating delicious and appetizing meals on keto.

REMEMBER

Preparation is the key to success. Dust off your stove and search your pantry shelves to get creative with healthy keto meals to keep you satisfied.

Snacking without Blowing Your Diet

We all do it, but keto dieters do it less. As you begin to eat more fat and a moderate amount of protein, you'll notice that you don't get as hungry in between meals. As you slash carbs, you'll also lose its addicting hold, as well as the rollercoaster highs and lows of blood sugar levels and won't feel the "hangry" urge to snack as much.

However, it's okay to eat a snack if you're not quite able to get to your next meal on time or as you're transitioning to keto and you still have some cravings.

Snacking in moderation

As mentioned, keto does not rely on snacking. Some people will eat every four or so hours, others may delay food up to six hours, and still others who intermittently fast may need to pack in their calories within six- or eight-hour windows and may seem like they're eating continuously during that time. Either way, a satisfying meal tends to be better for your gut health, letting your digestive system rest and recuperate in between meals. Just like your muscles, your gut needs rest to do some housecleaning, so in the hours that you aren't eating, your gut is cleaning up, getting rid of bacteria, and making preparations for its next meal. If you constantly snack, the system can get clogged up, leading to gut issues.

If you do choose to snack, do so because you're hungry, not for social reasons and definitely not out of boredom. The keto diet allows you to really tune into your body's hunger cues and bring mindfulness to your eating. Because you don't have mindless carb cravings (or won't within a few weeks, if you just started!), you can really check in to see if you're truly hungry or if your mind is just wandering. If you find yourself reaching for a snack out of boredom, stop, redirect, and find other ways to relieve your boredom and make better use of your time.

Keeping the carbs at bay

A host of low-carb snacking options are available to the keto dieter. You don't have to rely on sugary treats or high-carb foods to tide you over. Instead, choose high-fat, moderate-protein foods that will satisfy you until you make it to your next meal. As the keto diet has become more popular, there is an increasing supply of keto-friendly snacks in packaged form, making things more convenient. However, processed foods, keto or not, have a ton of fillers that may not be so healthy.

Try to focus on minimally processed whole foods, even when you snack, which will save you from the litany of preservatives and artificial sugars found in packaged "snack foods."

Great low-carb, whole-food keto options include

>> Nuts and seeds

>> Eggs

>> Keto-friendly smoothies

>> Veggies with nut butter

>> Fat bombs (a combination of nut/coconut butter, coconut oil, and your flavor of choice)

REMEMBER

A lot of seemingly appropriate snacks, like jerkies with maple glaze, may have hidden carbs. If you choose a packaged meal, make sure to inspect the nutrition label closely.

Replenishing Lost Fluids and Electrolytes

Glucose and glycogen (from carbs) retain water, and getting rid of these is often a dehydrating experience if you're not intentionally drinking quite a bit of water to compensate. Drinking water throughout the day is essential. As your insulin levels drop and carb storage plummets, you'll lose water that is typically attached to your liver and muscles' carb stores. You can easily replace this lost water, as long as you remember to drink throughout the day. You lose a lot of water daily through breathing, urinating, and sweat, so it's important to stay hydrated.

Drinking plenty of water

On average, you lose about 500 milliliters of water through breathing and between 1 and 2 liters through urination. Living in a humid and hot climate or exercising will bump up the fluids (and electrolytes) lost through sweating. You have to replace all that precious water to be at your best.

TIP

Here are some simple hacks to keep your water intake up to par:

>> Get a large water bottle and mark equally spaced lines on the side with times to hold you accountable for the amount of water you to drink through the day.

>> Set a timer to drink water every two hours.

>> Keep a large glass of water by your bedside and drink it as soon as you get up each morning.

Restoring your electrolytes

Whenever you lose water (especially through sweat), you're also losing valuable electrolytes. You have to replenish these minerals throughout the day. You get electrolytes from food, but you'll need additional minerals, especially during your transition to keto. People eating keto may need more salt than the average person on a high-carb diet because they're prone to excess sodium loss. A simple way to combat this is to opt for bone and veggie broths, become a little more liberal with the salt shaker, or drink electrolyte water to meet your needs. You'll notice if you've lost too many electrolytes because you'll feel weak, and you may experience headaches and lightheadedness.

Here are the key electrolytes to fuel up on:

>> **Salt (sodium chloride):** The main electrolyte in your body, salt goes with water to ensure that water is spread out through your body optimally. Salt is also vital for essential electrical gradients (yes, your body is electrical) that make sure your cells work at their best. Low salt levels will leave you feeling dizzy, tired, and lightheaded.

>> **Potassium:** Potassium is the next most common electrolyte in your body. It tends to stay inside your cells (rather than on the outside of the cells, like salt), and it's also critical in keeping the electrical gradient of your body up to par. Potassium is vital for muscle contraction, both of your large skeletal muscles that are working when you do a bench press, and of your steadily ticking heart. Low levels of potassium can lead to muscle weakness, stomach issues, and even abnormal heart rhythms.

>> **Magnesium:** This electrolyte is a workhorse that is critical in many areas of your body. It's needed in more than 300 different processes. Magnesium helps with many of the necessary enzymatic reactions that produce energy in your body. It plays a role in muscle contractions, as well as optimal nerve function and maintaining strong bones. Low magnesium levels can lead to muscle spasms, weakness, and fatigue, as well as nausea and vomiting. It's vital to replace this electrolyte, especially if you're going through keto flu.

>> **Calcium:** Although most people only think of calcium as the mineral that keeps bones healthy, it's also a vital nutrient that supports nerve and muscle function, as well as a component of the pathways that allows blood to clot. Low calcium levels are primarily associated with weak bones and teeth.

>> **Phosphate:** This essential mineral is vital for energy production, as well as cell function and bone strength. It's rare to be deficient in phosphate, but if it happens, you can expect bone pain and muscle weakness.

TIP

Make a point to stay hydrated and add vital electrolytes back into your diet as you transition to keto. It will make a noticeable difference in your energy levels.

Chapter **8**

Making Sure You're Getting the Nutrition You Need

When you start the keto diet, you'll need to brush up on proper nutrition. Many people still think keto means bacon and cheese, or hamburgers without buns, but keto is more than just protein and fat. Keto involves high-quality ingredients that are hard to come by in your local fast food restaurant. Often, these food establishments choose omega-6 heavy cooking oils that keto shuns, and are weak on nutritious, low-carb veggies that are filled with the vitamins, fiber, and antioxidants needed on the keto diet. Additionally, this misconception often overemphasizes the protein aspect of keto, mistaking it for a high-protein diet.

As you learn more about keto, you'll realize the difference between "dirty" keto and nutritious, whole-food "keto." Dirty keto looks at the macros only, primarily emphasizing the very low number of carbs but not evaluating the source of calories. With whole-food keto, it's important to make sure the carbs you do get are high in fiber, while the fats and proteins are high in antioxidants, medium-chain triglycerides (MCTs), and omega-3s to ensure that you get all the benefits of going keto.

Counting Net Carbs, Not Total Carbs

As we mention in Chapter 1, there are three different types of carbs, only two of which you need to stay away from:

>> Complex carbohydrates (starch)

>> Simple carbohydrates (sugar)

The third type of carbohydrate — indigestible carbohydrates (or fiber) — is actively encouraged.

Classic examples of carbohydrates are whole-grain pasta (starch), sodas (sugars), and psyllium husks, the main ingredient in Metamucil (fiber). We hope you're fully aware by now that starch and sugars are mostly forbidden, while fiber is a necessary part of keto. Starchy foods often contain fiber, but there are many other non-starch sources of fiber, so you don't have to blow your ketosis to get the recommended amounts. Because the body can't digest fiber, it doesn't absorb it or use it as glucose, making it perfect for the keto lifestyle.

Total carbohydrates are simply the sum total of all carbohydrates you consume, but they aren't what you should count for keto. *Net carbohydrates* are what you have when you subtract all carbs from fiber and other non-digestible carbs; this latter group is usually referred to as "other carbs" on a nutrition label. These carbs most commonly consist of sugar alcohols, such as erythritol, sorbitol, and xylitol. Although these alcohols are derived from sugar, they aren't digested as such and don't raise your blood sugar, meaning they don't impact your ability to begin and remain in ketosis.

REMEMBER

Whenever you look at the total carbs on the nutritional labels, always subtract the fiber — it doesn't count toward your daily carb intake, and it's good for you, to boot!

TIP

All the recipes in this book list the total carbs and the net carbs — and you *know* they're keto friendly!

Curbing Your Protein Intake

REMEMBER

Protein can turn into glucose if you overdo it. Your body, and particularly your brain, requires a certain amount of glucose to operate, and although the majority of your energy needs are effectively met by ketones, this core element can't be replaced by anything else.

On the standard American diet, the brain uses about 120 grams of glucose per day. It's an energy hog — although the brain typically accounts for only 2 percent of your body weight, it consumes approximately 20 percent of the energy you use in any given day. Ketones can provide up to 75 percent of this nutritional requirement, but the rest has to be supplied by glucose. If you're on a very-low-carb diet, or even a no-carb diet, you may be wondering how these needs are supplied. Some critics use this as a reason to condemn keto, but this conclusion is incorrect. Our amazing bodies have developed a process called *gluconeogenesis,* so even these core needs can be met in a zero-carb environment.

TECHNICAL STUFF

Gluconeogenesis is when the body takes a molecule of either protein or fat and breaks it down into three fatty-acid chains and a molecule of glycerol. The fatty acids are used by the body to satisfy the other 80 percent of your body's needs, but they can't help the brain because fatty acids don't cross the blood–brain barrier. That's where the glycerol comes in: It's further converted in the body to glucose and used by the brain as fuel.

This is all great news, but like any process in the body, we can overdo it. Overconsumption of protein can lead to excess gluconeogenesis, meaning that you can potentially cause your body to overproduce glucose even if you're avoiding carbs like the plague. Critics of the ketogenic diet often discuss issues caused by high-protein diets and characterize keto as such, but this isn't the case. Keto is a high-fat, medium-protein, low-carb diet. You shouldn't be afraid of protein by any means — just know that it is possible to overdo your protein consumption.

Unless you're training for an Olympic event or you're already malnourished, it's best to stick to the standard proportion of protein and not go too much beyond 20 percent of your total caloric intake. Knowing the general amount of protein in each of your foods is a great way to start. If you look down at your plate and have no idea of the macros in anything, check out Chapter 23 for helpful resources and guides to figuring out macros in everyday foods on the keto diet. The lists will give you a good sense of what and how much protein you should be eating.

To get you started, here are the approximate grams of protein in some keto foods:

>> **Meat, fish, or chicken (3 ounces):** 24 grams

>> **Tofu (3 ounces):** 7 grams

>> **Tempeh (3 ounces):** 15 grams

>> **Full-fat yogurt, no added sugars (1 cup):** 15 grams

>> **One egg:** 7 grams

>> **Hard cheese (1 ounce):** 7 grams

>> **Nuts (1 ounce):** 5 to 7 grams

TIP

Three ounces of meat is about the size of a deck of cards, while the same amount of fish is about the size of a checkbook. One ounce of cheese is about the size of four dice, and a cup is about the size of a tennis ball. An ounce of almonds is about 22 nuts.

Going Full Fat, Skipping Low-Fat

We hate to belabor the point, but never, ever choose the low-fat option. Low fat may just as well be called "high carb," because when fat is removed, sugars are routinely added. Common culprits are fruit-flavored yogurts and low-fat baked goods. Turn the container around and check out the sugar content. If you're not shocked, you haven't been paying attention!

Food needs flavor, and fat is the way nature usually decides to meet this need. Unfortunately, during the low-fat craze of the 1990s, people moved away from this thought process and began to replace fat with sugar. Ironically, although this was an attempt at healthy eating, obesity rates skyrocketed, diabetes increased, and cardiovascular disease became more and more of a problem. As time went on, and doctors and scientists were able to observe the long-term effects of swapping fat for sugar, the verdict became clear: Excess sugar is a problem, and a diet high in fat is actually very beneficial for you.

Even in the case of plain (no added sugar) dairy products, full fat is still great for you. The USDA and other organizations have been on a mission to promote low-fat and nonfat products for years, encouraging people to stay away from the full-fat, creamier versions. However, these guidelines haven't always been based on complete scientific information. New research shows that full-fat dairy is good for you: In a study that followed almost 3,000 adults over 22 years, blood levels of fatty acids found in full-fat dairy products did not increase the risk of heart disease and stroke at all. One of the fatty acids, heptadecanoic acid, actually decreased chances of dying from heart disease. Besides, full-fat dairy has MCT (like coconut oil), which decreases triglyceride levels and increases high-density lipoprotein (HDL) cholesterol (the "good" kind). This goes against decades of advice to stay away from these good-for-you fats. So, enjoy that extra dollop of cream!

REMEMBER

Full-fat foods have benefits that are skimmed away in the low-fat varieties. Despite the overarching concerns about weight gain and heart disease, research shows that full fat actually helps decrease all these ills. Choose the full-fat option whenever possible.

Replenishing Your Electrolytes

If you're feeling low in energy, fatigued, or just plain run down on keto, the problem may be a loss of electrolytes. You'll lose more of these valuable minerals on keto, so you have to be prepared to continuously replenish them. The most important electrolytes are sodium, potassium, magnesium, and calcium — they also include simple salts, such as sodium chloride.

Electrolytes are fascinating substances. Because the body is electrical in nature (shocking, we know), chemicals such as sodium and potassium form electrically charged particles called *ions* in body fluids and ensure our body processes are functioning normally. In addition to the symptoms we mention earlier, one of the most commonly seen symptoms of electrolyte loss is cramps. Cramps occur when a muscle misfires, contracting when it isn't supposed to. When you're missing these ions, your body begins to malfunction in odd and random ways. Think of them like you would motor oil in a car: It's not what makes the car run, but without it, it's definitely what makes the car stop.

Although most people think of Gatorade, a banana, or coconut water as the optimal way to replace electrolytes, these high-sugar options will immediately kick you out of ketosis. In addition to electrolyte water and sugar-free drinks (see Chapter 6), there are several other ways to keep your mineral levels up on keto. Here are some great options:

>> Fermented veggies (such as sauerkraut, kimchi, or pickles)

>> Avocados

>> Nut butter slathered on low-carb veggies (celery is a great option)

Whatever you choose, make sure you're thinking about these valuable nutrients and checking the labels (some brands can have hidden sugars as ingredients). Be hyperaware if you live in a humid environment or exercise vigorously; both of these factors induce sweating, which is one of the primary ways you lose electrolytes from your system.

Adding Healthy Oils to Your Diet

We've already mentioned the great health benefits of oils and fats like olive oil and coconut oil. With their high levels of monounsaturated fatty acids (MUFAs) and MCTs, respectively, these oils are heart-healthy, decrease the risk of diabetes, and help you lose weight. Needless to stay, these should be staples in your pantry, and you'll likely be eating them every day on the keto diet.

However, if you're looking for other oils to add to your pantry, here are some great options for cold dishes:

>> **Avocado oil:** Like the avocado itself, its oil is another good source of MUFAs. Compared to its parent fruit, avocado oil has just a hint of buttery goodness, but it's otherwise quite bland, meaning it will absorb any of the seasonings you decide to add to it.

>> **Walnut oil:** This oil is high in the alpha-linolenic acid (ALA) variety of omega-3 fats, as well as heart-healthy MUFAs. It's highly anti-inflammatory, making it a good choice to decrease your risk of insulin resistance and improve your gut health. Make sure to keep it refrigerated, and use by the expiration date, because it can go bad relatively quickly.

>> **MCT oil:** The epicenter of coconut oil, MCTs provide all the benefits of coconut oil in concentrated form (coconut oil is only 50 percent MCT). MCT is a great option to help kick your body into ketosis as you initially transition, and it has a host of other benefits, like improving heart health and your cholesterol levels (both low-density lipoprotein [LDL] and HDL).

TIP

It's easy to add oils to your keto diet. Here are some of our favorite ways:

>> Make an oil-based marinade with your favorite herbs and spices — oregano, black pepper, and paprika are some great seasonings to try.

>> Make your own salad dressing with a base of olive oil.

>> Add coconut oil, ghee, or MCTs to your coffee or tea for a decadent latte.

>> Stir-fry some veggies and protein in coconut or olive oil for an easy and nutritious meal.

>> Make a "fat bomb" — a mix of coconut oil, nut butter, and keto-friendly flavorings of your choice.

Getting Enough Fiber

The Institute of Medicine recommends that women under 50 get about 25 grams of fiber and men under 50 get 38 grams. If you're over 50, the numbers decrease to 30 grams for men and 21 grams for women. Sadly, the average American only eats about 15 grams of fiber, so there is a lot of room for improvement.

There are two types of fiber:

>> **Soluble:** Dissolves in water and helps to reduce blood sugar spikes and improve cholesterol levels.

>> **Insoluble:** Doesn't dissolve in water and also helps with digestion. It's the one that helps bulk up your stool and can make a trip to the bathroom a little easier.

Although you can't digest the soluble fiber, your many friendly gut bacteria love to feed on the sugars in fiber, which does wonders for your gut health. These soluble fibers are called *prebiotics* because they nourish the *probiotics* (bacteria) that live in the gut. Prebiotics are nothing new — our prehistoric forefathers have been chomping on these healthy foods for millennia. Research shows that Paleolithic man probably ate about 135 grams per day of prebiotics — a far cry from what the modern American consumes in the course of a day.

Soluble fiber can convert to glucose through a process known as *intestinal gluconeogenesis* (IGN), which occurs when the fiber ferments in the gut. Because IGN generates glucose, people once believed that soluble fiber should be counted toward daily carb allotment. But multiple studies have indicated something completely different: It turns out that intestinal glucose actually *lowers* blood sugar levels, increasing insulin sensitivity and assisting the body in getting into ketosis.

There are four primary benefits of eating fiber:

>> **It slows the rate at which sugar is absorbed in the bloodstream.** Although this is less of a concern when your energy is being provided by ketones, it can make a crucial difference if you accidentally overindulge in carbs. Slowing the rate at which that glucose reaches the bloodstream moderates its effects, giving you a much higher chance of staying in ketosis.

>> **It moves through your intestines more quickly than other foods.** The benefits for regulating bowel movements are obvious, but there's another, hidden benefit to this fascinating fiber fact. Ghrelin is one of the crucial hunger-regulating hormones in the body and is produced in the gastrointestinal (GI) tract when it senses that you need to eat. When the brain receives these signals, it triggers a feeling of hunger, making you want to eat. Fiber speeds right to the source of ghrelin production, causing the body to stop producing it because it senses that you're full. You should always eat slowly and chew fully, and starting your meal with fiber will likely inhibit your appetite, making you feel fuller even when you're decreasing your caloric intake.

>> **It physically cleans your colon.** One of the challenges probiotic supplement-makers face, for example, is that so much is digested in the stomach that it can be difficult to get anything to the colon in a relatively intact state. Because insoluble fiber, in particular, can't be digested, it handles the trip to the intestines much better than most other foods. When it arrives, it physically scrubs the sides of your intestines as it moves through your system; this cleans out old bacteria and any old buildup in your system. Not only does this keep you regular, but studies have shown that it's a key contributing factor in reducing your chances of developing colon cancer.

>> **It keeps you regular.** We've mentioned this before in passing (pun intended), but it bears repeating. One of the more commonly complained-about side effects of keto is constipation (see Chapter 10 for more detail), and fiber is a critical component of fighting and eliminating this pesky issue. As you transition to a fat-based diet and reduce your calories slightly (not drastically), you're causing your body to feed off of its fat reserves, which means you'll be generating less solid waste. You'll likely find that your bowel movements are smaller and less frequent, but that also means you may have to work harder to pass them if you're not staying hydrated and consistently consuming an appropriate amount of fiber. Two common names for insoluble fiber are "roughage" and "bulk"; you'll find that it's easier to pass waste if it's of a reasonable size, and fiber helps ensure this. Alternately, if you find yourself struggling with diarrhea, fiber will help bind stools together and eliminate further dehydration and discomfort.

Several common health concerns are addressed by increased fiber intake. The first is hemorrhoids, often triggered by spending too much time on the toilet or straining too hard to pass stools. Fiber lubricates everything in the GI tract, allowing things to pass quickly and efficiently, limiting your time on the throne.

Diverticular disease is an overarching term for a number of specific conditions that can affect your large intestine. When your colon isn't moving things along the way it should, your chances of experiencing this condition increase. Small bulges, or *sacs*, form on the side walls of the colon and create the risk of being perforated or torn. This can lead to nasty infections, surgery, and potentially severe complications. The best way to deal with any kind of diverticular disease is to avoid it in the first place, and the starting point for prevention is consistent fiber consumption.

Keto-approved vegetables that are high in fiber include

>> Artichokes

>> Asparagus

>> Bell peppers

- » Broccoli
- » Brussels sprouts
- » Cabbage
- » Cauliflower
- » Cucumber
- » Green beans
- » Radishes
- » Spinach
- » Zucchini

You can also find keto-friendly fruits that are high in fiber:

- » Avocados
- » Blackberries
- » Coconut
- » Lemons
- » Limes
- » Olives
- » Raspberries
- » Strawberries
- » Tomatoes

REMEMBER

Fiber is the ultimate free carb!

Inulin is a prebiotic fiber that is good for you. Studies show that inulin can help to improve the ability to absorb calcium and magnesium, likely increasing bone health, while other studies suggest that inulin may help to reduce cholesterol levels in the blood, increasing our heart health.

Some keto-friendly foods that contain high amounts of inulin are

- » **Nuts:** These can come with up to 9 grams of fiber in a 1-cup serving.
- » **Asparagus:** Three ounces of asparagus provide nearly 3 grams of fiber.
- » **Cauliflower:** This keto-friendly substitute for mashed potatoes or pizza crust can provide up to 3 grams of fiber for every cup.

» **Garlic:** Three ounces of this flavorful bulb can provide you with 16 grams of fiber. This more than makes up for the garlic breath.

» **Onions:** You can get up to 3 grams of fiber for every cup of onions you eat.

» **Tempeh:** This fermented soy food provides a substantial amount of fiber — up to 7 grams of fiber for every ½ cup serving.

TIP

Many people don't eat enough fiber on a daily basis. This can lead to unfortunate gut issues both in the long term and in the short term that can make adopting a keto lifestyle a challenge. Take charge of your gut health by including high-fiber foods in your diet.

Chapter **9**

Eating Out and Loving It!

I f you barely know how to boil an egg, an exciting part of the keto lifestyle is that it can build your confidence in the kitchen! Learning how to marinate, grill, and sauté will have you looking forward to the question "What's for dinner?" like never before. Knowing that your time and energy went into preparing your meal also provides a sense of satisfaction and increased enjoyment when you sit down to eat it. Eating at home gives you valuable control of knowing exactly what you're putting into your body and where it comes from. You'll never get that satisfaction from eating out where there are always "secret sauces" or questionable food practices.

However, you may want to give your cooking skills a night off occasionally, and eating out on the keto diet shouldn't provoke anxiety. After all, eating out usually brings up images of decadent and satisfying food, and that will be your mode of operation on keto. Still, it's essential to be aware that many people equate high carbs with decadence, so make sure to stay clear of these practices. With a little foresight and insightful questioning, you'll enjoy dining out on occasion.

Choosing Keto-Friendly Restaurants

There are a host of restaurants that will have something satisfying and low-carb for you to enjoy during your meal out. Although you may need to tweak a thing or two, many restaurants will be well-prepared for customers who choose a keto lifestyle and will happily make a swap from high-carb foods to something that will fit into your diet. More and more restaurants are beginning to boast a "low-carb" section of the menu that will help take the guesswork out of ordering.

TIP

It's a good idea take a couple of moments to check the restaurant's online menu to get a sense of the lay of the (food) land. This way, before you sit down to your meal, you'll be prepared with a few ideas about what to choose, as well as the questions you'll need to have answered before ordering. Many restaurants include a modest list of the ingredients in the entrées so you can identify if it fits into your lifestyle. Scoping out the menu gives you a chance to see how keto-friendly the restaurant really is, as well as important characteristics like sensitivity to dietary concerns (such as gluten-free options) and food quality (such as grass-fed beef and organic fare).

There are a few things you should always avoid. Regular soft drinks are iconic pairs with many restaurant dishes, but they pack on the carbs unbelievably quickly. An average soft drink contains 39 grams of sugar, or nearly 10 teaspoons per glass! If you're from the South, you're familiar with the delicious treat known as sweet tea — unfortunately, it has at least as much sugar as a Coke or Pepsi. Water is a safe go-to, and you can ask for your server to bring lemons to add a bit of flavor. Ask for other carb-free options, such as diet soda or sugar-free lemonade.

Potatoes are another popular item that come in more forms than you can count; unfortunately, they're off the menu. Many restaurants, including fast-food fare, offer salads, however, so trade in those spuds for spinach!

Steakhouses and barbeque

These restaurants are a keto lover's dream. You'll have a lot of different fatty beef prepared in numerous ways, as well as options for seafood and chicken if you choose. Go to town on a ribeye steak and enjoy it with extra butter or creamy sauce with some roasted veggies. You may have to skip some of the barbecue sauce because they often have added sugar (usually honey or brown sugar). Also, stay away from all types of fries, as well as any sugar-filled desserts.

Generally speaking, you'll want to avoid anything that's been breaded, because this is a significant source of hidden carbohydrates. Ordering a side Caesar salad is a great choice, but make sure that they hold the croutons! Coleslaw is a popular side at barbeque joints and is typically very keto-friendly; just ask if they've added any unique ingredients that may challenge your macros.

If you're in the mood for a burger, you're in luck! This traditional American fare has a very keto-friendly base, but you'll want to avoid the bun, ketchup, and any kind of barbecue sauce. Most restaurants are happy to replace the bread with a lettuce wrap, saving valuable carbs from your daily allowance. If you like mustard, however, feel free to go to town! Other traditional hamburger toppings like lettuce, tomatoes, onions, and pickles are usually great options for keto.

Buffets

You should be able to find a host of options at buffets because they're based on diversity. You can choose grilled or roasted meat or poultry, as well as salads and steamed or grilled veggies. Choose an oil-based vinaigrette over the low-fat or fruity-flavored salad dressings. Sometimes, you'll need to ask them to bring out these options, but most restaurants have them. Choose egg-based dishes if it's time for brunch. Stay away from most fried meats because they'll likely have a breading or flour coating, adding unwanted carbs to your meal.

One solid strategy is to leave "breathing room" on your plate. Mimic the portions you would have at home, knowing you can always make a second trip if you like. Studies have repeatedly shown that the more food we put on our plates, the more we eat; forcing yourself to make several trips will help dial those calories down and help you make better, more intentional choices each time. Start off with a salad, then make a second trip for your entrée.

REMEMBER

A crucial element to controlling portion size is the speed at which you eat. If you chow down quickly, your body's hormones lag behind your intake, and you end up overeating and feeling stuffed and miserable. That food isn't going anywhere, so take your time — enjoy the company of your family or friends and the atmosphere, putting as much effort into conversation as you are into chewing!

Seafood

Seafood is a great option. You'll get your fill of omega-3s with hearty, fatty fish. You can choose crustaceans like shrimp, lobster, and crabs, which are often lower in carbs than mollusks. Make sure you don't get any deep-fried breaded options like calamari. Salmon is also always a great option because it's high in protein and heart-healthy omega-3s, as well as a host of vitamins and minerals. Choose seasonal grilled or steamed veggies as your side. Ask for extra butter or a cream-based sauce to make it a true keto dream.

As a general rule, any of the fish or crustaceans on the menu are keto-approved. What isn't is the breading that often accompanies them. Crab that's been drenched in butter, for example, is a fantastic dish you should have no qualms about chowing down on. Crab cakes, however, are loaded with carbs and need to be on the "no-go" list.

Dishes that are advertised as "fresh" or "pan-fried" are better options than anything that's been deep-fried. On the off-chance that you actually find something deep-fried that isn't smothered in breading, it's still prepared in the same oil that all the other breaded dishes go through and could be a source of a significant number of hidden carbs.

Many restaurants pair seafood with pasta; as appetizing as it looks, both the pasta and the sauce that accompanies it are normally out of bounds for ketoers. Thankfully, any place that offers noodles often places as much of an emphasis on salads as they do the traditional Italian offerings, so flip over to that section of the menu and have at it!

Mediterranean

Mediterranean food may have some of the best options available for heart health, with an easy choice to slather extra-virgin olive oil on virtually everything you eat. This is also one of the broadest genres of dining fare: Mediterranean food pulls offerings from Greek, Italian, Spanish, Algerian, Libyan, Moroccan, Lebanese, Syrian, Turkish, and Israeli dishes. These wide-ranging culinary approaches have a few things in common. One is a heavy emphasis on olive oil, which should pique any keto dieter's interest. Fresh vegetables and a wide range of healthy cheeses, both hard and soft, are also typically seen in this type of cuisine. One aspect of Mediterranean dining is that, although fresh breads and pita are a staple, they're rarely combined in the ways you see in American fare. Carbs here are often served as stand-alone offerings, making them easy to exclude from your plate.

Most Mediterranean restaurants will have fresh fish and seafood available, as well as options for lamb or chicken. You can also enjoy low-carb seasonal veggies like peppers, tomatoes, cucumbers, and spinach. Opt for a side salad or grilled vegetables over starchy options like gyros or breaded foods. Make sure to squeeze lemon on your fish or salad and benefit from the herbs used in Mediterranean spices like mint, oregano, and garlic for extra flavor and antioxidants. Choose right, and you'll get healthy fats filled with monounsaturated fatty acids (MUFAs) and omega-3s.

One potentially surprising element of Mediterranean dining is the health benefits introduced by vinegar, which is a staple of this kind of food. Vinegar improves insulin sensitivity and assists in weight loss efforts. It also suppresses appetite and delays the speed at which sugar enters your bloodstream.

Japanese

Japanese food tends to be high in fresh seafood, as well as fermented foods like miso and pickled seaweed salad or ginger. These are great options.

Rice is a huge component of Japanese dining, and this is off-limits for keto. You'll also want to avoid the edamame; ½ cup of these delicious soybeans contain about 9 grams of carbs! If you're a fan of seaweed salad, beware that although the base is very healthy, it's usually flavored with a variety of flavor-inducing agents that tend to be pretty high in sugar.

TIP

Focus on the sashimi rather than the sushi menu to avoid rice, or ask if they're willing to make rolls with only seaweed wrapping (some will!). If you'd rather not eat raw food, choose the yakitori, which includes grilled meats and veggies. Make sure to stay away from tempura (deep fried and breaded), as well as teriyaki sauces, which tend to have a lot of sweeteners. Instead, ask for miso soup or tamari/soy sauce for flavoring. If you enjoy ramen, you can always ask them to skip the noodles and enjoy a hearty pork broth with all the extra meat, egg, mushroom, and green onions you want.

If you can find it, Konjac ramen is an excellent choice. Unlike traditional ramen noodles, Konjac is made from the root of the elephant yam and is very low-carb (typically 3 grams per 100 grams of noodles).

As far as drink options go, green tea is an excellent option and widely available. If you feel like going for a more adult beverage, sake is on the approved list, but beer tacks on the carbohydrates quickly.

Chinese

Chinese food can be a great option, as long as you stay away from many of the sauces that will be sweetened with sugars or have hidden thickening agents like potato starches; these can dramatically increase your carb intake without your realizing it. Choose chicken, beef, or tofu options without these added sauces. Instead, opt for steamed or roasted options, as well as fatty cuts of meats like pork belly. Good choices are egg foo young, steamed pork ribs, roasted duck, and steamed veggies like bok choy and broccoli.

Many Chinese dishes are deep-fried — avoid these because the same oil has likely been used to fry every dish with breading, even if what you ordered is (allegedly) virtually carb-free. The upside of this is that steamed food is nearly as popular, presenting a much healthier set of choices. Steamed fish, tofu, and vegetables shouldn't be difficult to find.

When considering soups and sauces, choose any options that are thinner and clearer, such as egg drop soup, rather than thick liquids that are almost certainly loaded with sugar and/or cornstarch. Sauces you should avoid include sweet and sour, hoisin, duck sauce, plum sauce, and oyster sauce — these sauces are loaded with extra sugar.

Traditional Chinese dishes that employ savory over sugary additives, however, include chicken with mushrooms, curry chicken, moo goo gai pan, and Szechuan prawns. Stir-fried dishes often have some cornstarch, but not nearly as much as those that have been prepared by deep-frying; if you're dining at a traditional restaurant rather than a buffet, you can ask if the chef will leave the starch out of your stir-fry. Walnut chicken is another favorite dish that is traditionally made without sugar or starch.

TIP

If you eat at a Chinese restaurant, just say no to hoisin, plum, oyster, or sweet-and-sour sauces.

Steering Clear of Carbs

In this section, we remind you of foods that have a hefty dose of carbs. Some (like bread, potatoes, and rice) are obvious, but you may be surprised at how many carbs condiments pack on to your otherwise keto-friendly food. Make sure to check with your server if any of these can be removed or replaced with keto-friendly alternatives:

>> **Bread and breading:** Let your server know that you don't want the bread basket. It's easy to be aware of the carbs in bread, but make sure to ask your server how a dish is prepared. You don't want to be surprised when your chicken comes out smothered in crispy breading. Many restaurants offer alternatives, like substituting grilled chicken for fried.

>> **Potatoes:** Skip potatoes in any form, including roasted, boiled, or fried. They're easily broken down into sugar in your blood. Unfortunately, this means no sweet potato fries as well; although they're more nutritious than white potatoes, sweet potatoes (especially baked varieties) have an extremely high glycemic index — as high as 94! — and are not a healthier choice in that regard. They have more nutrients, but also higher amounts of carbs.

>> **Rice:** This includes all types, including brown, black, and wild varieties. All varieties of rice have almost exactly the same glycemic index and will cause unwanted blood sugar spikes and insulin resistance over time. Ask that your main dish is put on a bed of greens rather than rice.

>> **Noodles and pasta:** These are completely off-limits. All pasta varieties, even those that are gluten-free or egg-based, are very high in carbs. An average 3-ounce serving — which most restaurants will at least double — has around 100 grams of carbs. Don't choose any pasta-based dishes. ***Remember:*** You're "pasta" all that!

>> **Sweet and starchy sauces and condiments:** All these condiments have varying amounts of added sugars and are often high in preservatives to boot. Many of them are also thickened with cornstarch, flour, or other carb-heavy thickening agents. These quickly add up.

>> **Balsamic vinegar:** Although vinegar provides a tremendous number of health benefits, this particular variety has the highest amount of carbs of the group. You'd be better served by choosing a lighter variety, such as white wine vinegar.

>> **Barbecue sauce:** A central ingredient of these sauces is brown sugar or molasses. These kinds of sauces are some of the most sugary available. It's definitely a poor choice for the keto lifestyle. Occasionally, you can find a barbecue sauce that's low in sugar, but if you do, it will certainly be advertised as such.

>> **Black bean sauce:** This sauce contains cornstarch, which adds to the overall carb load. Don't choose this — overindulging can help to push you out of ketosis.

>> **Ketchup:** Surprisingly, most ketchup is filled with high fructose corn syrup, even though it's not particularly sweet. We were surprised to find that 2 tablespoons of the stuff contains the same amount of carbs as a glass of milk. It's best to skip the ketchup altogether. Similar to barbecue sauce, you *can* find low- or no-sugar ketchup options; if you do, however, it will certainly be advertised as such.

>> **Sriracha:** A key component of this sauce is brown sugar, so it's definitely not carb free. If you love this spicy flavor, though, never fear — the makers of sriracha also make a sugar-free version of it. You can ask your server if the restaurant carries this. Or better yet, order it on Amazon and carry it around with you wherever you go!

>> **Teriyaki:** This sauce packs on the sweeteners — using both honey and brown sugar — and also uses cornstarch as a thickener. It's not a good idea to eat anything that is covered in this sauce.

>> **Sweet salad dressings:** Always stay away from the low-fat salad dressings or the fruit-flavored varieties. These condiments are loaded with carbs because they're filled with sweeteners.

>> **Most desserts:** Few restaurants offer keto-friendly desserts, so just skip the dessert menu altogether. Instead, you can ask for a cheese plate, depending on the type of restaurant you're in. Or ask for a dish of berries (not all types of fruit) if you want to splurge on your carbs for the day.

TIP

Choose unsweetened condiments like mayonnaise, horseradish sauce, mustard (but not honey mustard), hot sauce, soy sauce, and *pico de gallo*. Use red or white wine vinegar instead of balsamic.

Loading Up on Fats and Proteins

Fats and proteins will be the basis of all your meals at restaurants. Eating out is supposed to be a luxury, so make sure you indulge in the wonderful fatty options available to you. Clearly let your server know that you are not afraid of extra fat. Look for these great options:

>> **Meats:** Choose the fattier cut of meat and don't be afraid of pork belly or duck, which are higher in fat.

>> **Seafood:** Eat the whole fish — the skin often has most of the omega-3s and helps seal in the nutrients as it's cooked. However, the skin may contain more of the toxins, like mercury, than other parts of the fish. Be sure to do your research and ask your server where the restaurant gets its fish. For example, one-third of the fish caught off of New Jersey shores have levels of mercury that are higher than recommended, and certain fish from the Gulf of Mexico should also be avoided.

>> **Low-carb veggies:** Pile these on, whether fried, steamed, grilled, or incorporated into a keto dish. Double-check with your waiter — mixed vegetables may have high-carb fares like carrots and corn. Some restaurants will happily switch to low-carb veggies if you ask, but be aware that others will have a premix sample of vegetables already prepared. It's seldom worth it to dig out carb-heavy ingredients while you try to enjoy your meal.

>> **Eggs:** Eggs are a key component of keto eating. There are a million ways to eat eggs, so enjoy the many options available to you.

>> **Cheese:** Choose hard cheeses like cheddar, gouda, parmesan, and pecorino. These have less lactose — and carbs — than softer varieties.

>> **Creamy sauces:** Cream-based sauces are a must on the keto diet. Pour them onto your cut of meat or over veggies, or add a dollop to soup. Be aware, however, that some cream-based sauces are thickened with flour. Ask your server to be sure, and skip these if he indicates that flour or cornstarch were used in their preparation.

>> **Butter and oils:** Always ask for a side of butter or oil for your meat and veggies. Most restaurants have an abundance of it in the kitchen and will happily fulfill your request.

Making Special Requests

You need to be vocal when you eat out. It's okay to make requests, and most restaurants will work with you to turn yours into reality. Always ask for clarification if you aren't sure what's in a specific sauce or how a food is prepared. Don't get stuck eating extra carbs you didn't want or only drinking water because you can't find anything on the menu.

Here are some tips for making requests in restaurants:

>> **Replace starches with veggies.** Most restaurants will be happy to replace rice, potatoes, or fries with a side salad or even grilled or roasted vegetables. Just ask.

>> **Replace gravy or sauces with butter or cream.** Gravies often have flour added, and sauces are often loaded with sugars and thickening agents. Ask your servers if they have more keto-friendly options. If they don't have any suggestions, merely ask for a small dish of butter or a dollop of cream.

These are also good choices to keep your carb intake low, while adding fat to your meal:

>> **Mayonnaise:** Oil and egg yolks definitely fill the fat quotient for keto. Feel free to plop it on top of your grilled veggies or fish or use it as a salad dressing. The options with mayo are virtually endless.

>> **Guacamole:** Based on the keto staple avocado, guacamole adds a tangy spiciness. Add it to your eggs or as a dip for veggies, or eat it by the mouthful if it suits your fancy. There's so much to love about guacamole!

>> **Hollandaise sauce:** The classic dressing of eggs Benedict, this is one of the most delicious sauces anyone could dream up, which is why the French did it. The sauce is a mix of egg yolks, melted butter, and lemon juice. It makes anything taste better, so feel free to add it to grilled or steamed veggies, drizzle it over your entrée, or just stare at it lovingly.

>> **Béarnaise sauce:** An offshoot of Hollandaise sauce, this creamy sauce has the same base, but it adds in an expert combination of spices to bring it all together. Although it's traditionally used as a sauce for steak, we love it on any protein and it's also a great dipping sauce for grilled veggies.

>> **Buffalo sauce:** This is a surprisingly good sauce for low-carb dieters. It doesn't have any hidden sugars, with less than 1 gram of carbs in a 1.5-ounce serving. It's typically made with butter, so it has a good amount of fat as well. Feel free to slather this all over your chicken wings!

Here are some other swaps you should get familiar with:

>> **Order blue cheese or vinegar and oil salad dressing.** Blue cheese is an excellent choice to top your salad, adding rich flavor and texture. Many restaurants will also provide an oil dispenser filled with olive oil. Ask for this and make sure they have red or white wine vinegar, rather than balsamic, which has more carbs.

>> **Convert your burger or sandwich into a lettuce wrap.** Many restaurants are happy to do this. You may even be aware of "secret menus" that already endorse "protein-style" options for burgers. If you're in a less casual restaurant, you can just ask your server to put the meat on a bed of greens and eat it like an open-faced sandwich.

>> **Drop the side dishes.** Let your server know that you won't want any starches and ask him or her what low-carb options are available as an alternative. Most restaurants will swap the fries for veggies or a small side salad that you can load up with your vinegar and oil dressing. If they won't accommodate this, just skip the sides altogether — then take note and don't return.

Ordering Keto by Meal: A Few Suggestions

If you find yourself at a restaurant and feel like there are no keto options, take a deep breath and look again. There are often minor changes you can make by swapping a side or adding some extra butter or oil to make lackluster food more appealing. Although this approach can be a major challenge when you first start out on the keto diet, there are several tricks we've cultivated over the past few years depending on different times of the day you find yourself at a new restaurant.

Here are a few options that should work well, regardless of what style of restaurant you choose.

Breakfast

TIP

Getting breakfast or brunch at a restaurant and not sure what you can eat? Choose eggs: It's the easiest and most versatile option, and almost any restaurant will have eggs as an option during the morning hours. With eggs, you'll get choline, fat–soluble vitamins, protein, and a host of other nutrients. Stay away from egg substitutes or egg whites that lack the nutrients and fat found in the yolk.

Good egg options include

>> **Scrambled eggs or an omelet with veggies:** Make sure the veggies are of the low-carb variety.

>> **Frittata:** Similar to a crustless quiche, this breakfast item often comes crammed with a variety of low-carb veggies, meats, and cheeses to provide a well-balanced meal.

>> **Eggs Benedict:** This American classic includes multiple sources of fat and protein to start your day off right. The Hollandaise sauce adds a flair of decadence to the meal. Make sure to skip the muffin it often comes with, and ask to have it placed on a bed of spinach instead.

Feel free to add a side of bacon, ham, or steak (if you're at a steakhouse), while skipping the hash browns.

If you're feeling tired of eggs, there's nothing wrong with bucking the trend and choosing dinner for breakfast, instead of the other way around.

Lunch

Lunch is a great time to choose a salad as a meal. Salads are the perfect keto meal because they're a great way to mix together your favorite protein and low-carb veggies with a hefty dose of healthy fats. Whether you prefer chicken, fish, steak, or even tofu as your protein source, make sure to hold croutons, wontons, dried fruit, and the low-fat salad dressings. Instead, pile on the nuts, seeds, and full-fat ranch dressing or oil and vinegar substitutes.

Another good choice is a lettuce wrap sandwich. Choose your go-to sandwich, and ask them to hold the bread. Instead, choose a lettuce wrap to keep everything together. Most restaurants will be happy to comply with your request. You can also choose to just eat the inside of the sandwich (or burrito) and leave the carbs behind if you're sure that you won't be tempted to eat some of the bread.

Dinner

Choose an entrée based on a good quality protein, like chicken, beef, pork, or seafood. Choose any variety that is grilled, broiled, or steamed. If you want to splurge, order the seasonal fish of the day, Kobe beef, or the duck. Then have a side of grilled or steamed veggies to finish things off.

If you can't find anything that looks like a tasty keto option, consider choosing a variety of appetizers for your meal. Many appetizers are good sources of protein and fat, so choosing several of these — and a vegetable side — is an excellent choice to keep you satisfied.

Soon after going keto we had to go on a work trip and were faced with eating out for almost every meal. Although initially, this felt like a recipe for disaster, we decided to rise to the occasion and find fun ways to make eating out on keto possible. The hotel we were staying at had the classic Italian-style restaurant of salad, pasta dishes, and pizza. After a couple of nights of eating large salads, we decided to get creative and make our own meals. We chose a plate of grilled, keto-friendly veggies; kebab-style meats; and an antipasti platter. The mix brought together bold flavors into a low-carb treat that we've chosen again and again when we eat Italian.

Opting for a Low-Sugar Beverage

The best bet when you go out is to drink water. Naturally carb-free, it's the top choice for staying hydrated and keeping you full and resistant to the sugar-sweetened desserts and carbs that are all too easy to indulge in at most restaurants.

Here are some great keto-friendly beverage options when you're eating out:

» **Water or sparkling water, with or without lemon:** The classic choice. You'll never go wrong with this refreshing liquid. Many restaurants are catching up with the infused water trend and may accommodate your request for a little extra flavor added to your water.

» **Coffee:** This is a valid option as an after-dinner treat or at a coffee shop. Drink it plain or add a splash of cream or half-and-half.

» **Tea:** Herbal, black, and green teas are good options. Most restaurants have multiple varieties and will be happy to provide more hot water. Make sure that if you choose an iced tea, it comes unsweetened.

» **Dry wines:** These tend to have about 4 grams of carbs per 5-ounce glass and are a good option if you're choosing to have some alcohol with your meal or you're out celebrating with friends and family.

» **Light beer:** This alcoholic option may have even fewer carbs than a glass of wine, depending on the brand. It's an excellent choice for a low-carb treat.

Dining at the Homes of Relatives or Friends

Socializing with friends and family is an integral part of life, and you should feel free to enjoy it regardless of your food choices. Socializing often comes with eating, but you don't have to jeopardize ketosis to do so. Try to be as transparent as possible about your food choices beforehand, and even offer to bring some yummy keto options if nothing will be available for you to eat.

Although some friends may feel a bit offended if you don't eat the food that they lovingly prepared, if you set clear boundaries and let them know that keto is crucial to you, they'll likely understand. Despite the concern, at a buffet-style affair or even at a sit-down dinner, there will be some proteins or fats that you can eat. Just steer clear of the carbs that surround them.

This was one of the hardest transitions for us. Our parents' homes are often filled with rice-based dishes, potatoes, and pastries. When we first mentioned that we were going keto, we were met with blank stares. When we explained that this meant no foods made from flour, they looked at us with abject horror. We may as well have mentioned that we were joining the circus. Over time, as we explained the reason for our choice, stuck to our guns, and backed it up with all the information we're sharing with you, our parents came around. Because there are also a lot of meat dishes and keto-friendly veggies, our parents just load us up with extra servings of these.

REMEMBER

Be honest and open with friends and family about your food preferences. When they see how important the keto lifestyle is to you, they'll likely be okay with your refusing the bread and potatoes. Offering to bring foods that are keto-friendly is a great way to be hospitable while making sure your own dietary needs are met.

Communicating your preferences

Discuss your preferences clearly and calmly. Casually mention that you're following the keto diet and making a choice to keep your carbs to a minimum. You don't need to give an hour-long lecture on the topic of keto, but let your friends and family know that it's important to you and it's a commitment to your health that you take seriously. Let them know that from now on you'll be skipping the rice and potatoes and, instead, will be asking for extra veggies with a side of butter.

Ask your host how he prepared the meal — or where it came from if it was catered. You'll learn a lot about how food is made, and you won't have to spend your time worrying about how many hidden carbs you may accidentally be consuming.

Here are some easy tips to clearly and politely communicate your preferences:

>> "That looks amazing, but I'm making a commitment to cut out foods high in carbohydrates for my health."

>> "No thanks, I don't want [whatever high-carb food], but I'd love an extra helping of these greens or meat [or another low-carb food]."

>> "It looks great, but I'd be happier with [a low-carb food]."

As you stay consistent and don't compromise on your preferences, friends and family will realize that you're committed to keto, and they'll be more receptive to honoring your choices. It's rare to have a loved one really opposed to keto, even if you may find that there may be a lot of misconceptions about the diet. Be patient, and most people will come around to your new eating habits.

TIP

Don't be shy about letting your preferences be known. It's better to be honest and let your hosts know why you aren't eating the food rather than risk miscommunication and being seen as snobbish, or worse.

Bringing your own beverage

Water is a great option that should always be available wherever you go for dinner. Always ask for it, even if you plan on drinking something else later. We've started carrying around electrolyte tablets wherever we go — they're easy to toss in a purse or have in your car — to add a little extra kick to water. You can bring this to your dinner party. Often, friends and family will want to try one because they're looking for ways to increase their water intake, too. Electrolyte water is an excellent idea if you're at a dinner party and the only other options are an array of juices or sodas.

If you're going to an event that you expect will include alcohol, offer to bring your favorite bottle of dry red or white wine that is keto-friendly. Even if your host offers cocktails, you can easily ask for seltzer water — or bring your own bottle of it — to make a more keto-friendly option. We've brought a can or two of Wave soda to add if we wanted a more flavorful option.

3
Overcoming Obstacles

Chapter **10**

Dealing with Undesirable Side Effects

Some lucky people sail right through the transition from the standard American diet to keto, but many people face a roadblock or two. The keto flu and specific issues like fatigue, dehydration, and constipation are common problems that accompany this major transition in eating. The trick is being prepared for these roadblocks so that if they occur, you aren't blindsided by intense fatigue, keto rash, or any other problems.

Keeping your focus on the long-term benefits can be difficult, but remember that the roadblocks we cover in this chapter are temporary and actually mean that your body is trying to adjust to positive changes you're making. These are the growing pains that will eventually carry you to the other side of the keto journey. In this chapter, we also fill you in on which changes suggest something is going wrong in your keto journey so you can correct course and move toward living your best life.

Getting Over the Hump: The Keto Flu

The keto flu is a common speed bump that, if it happens, will begin a few days into starting the keto journey. Keto flu is one of the most frequently experienced consequences of going keto, but it can be overcome quite easily if you're prepared with a few tricks up your sleeve. You'll know you are going through the keto flu if you have

>> Muscle aches and weakness

>> Brain fog and difficulty concentrating

>> Headaches

>> Intense fatigue

>> Insomnia

>> Gut issues like indigestion, constipation, and even diarrhea

REMEMBER

Your body is making a significant change in its basic mode of operation, and the keto flu and other symptoms are just signs that the kinks are getting worked out. As your glucose stores drop and your body turns to fat as the primary source of energy, the many genes, enzymes, and proteins needed to accomplish this goal must come out of hibernation and ramp up to do the job. Your body has to go through the transition period of getting used to these new processes before it can become efficient at using fat as fuel.

TIP

The first thing you'll need is patience. Your body is doing its best to keep up with your good intentions — give it time and remember to be gentle with yourself and your body. Make sure that you won't be preparing for a major exam, gearing up for an intense work deadline, or having a slew of social activities around the time of your keto transition. If you have a break from work or school, use that time to start the keto diet. Or, if you can't afford that luxury, at least make sure it's at a time of relative calm in your life. You need to remove as many obstacles as you can to ensure you stay on keto; trying to completely change your eating style while going through other life transitions or periods of stress can be overwhelming.

If you don't have any downtime to transition, or you're trying to go keto a second or third time because of roadblocks in the past, a good suggestion is to slowly decrease your carb intake instead of jumping headfirst into a diet where you're suddenly restricted to 25 grams of carbs per day. You'll still get to ketosis if your journey takes a little longer. If you're on the standard American diet, you're likely consuming 150 to 200 grams of carbs per day; over a few weeks, slowly drop down to less than 50 grams of carbs per day. This will help decrease your risk of going through severe keto flu.

If you do end up experiencing symptoms of keto flu, you can decrease the severity — or eliminate it altogether — by following a few simple steps. In no particular order, here are our top five remedies to get you through the keto flu:

>> **Take an Epsom salt bath.** Epsom salts are magnesium sulfate crystals, and they're great for relaxing sore muscles and decreasing pain. We recommend putting 1 or 2 cups of Epsom salts in a warm (not scalding) bath and soaking for at least 20 minutes. For an added benefit, choose a lavender and Epsom salt combo or add a few drops of lavender oil to your bath. Lavender is also known for its ability to relieve tight muscles and will add a relaxing and soothing quality to your experience.

>> **Eat (and drink) your minerals (salt, potassium, and magnesium).** You can quickly lose salt and potassium on the ketogenic diet, so it's vital that you replace them. Losing these essential minerals can cause the symptoms of keto flu, so if you replace them before they get too low, you may save yourself a challenging few days. Additionally, magnesium helps mitigate symptoms like constipation and muscle aches. To replenish these lost minerals, drink electrolyte water or bone or vegetable broth, and eat potassium-rich foods like avocado. Another good option is to take a potassium and magnesium supplement during your transition and get friendly with the salt shaker.

>> **Stay hydrated.** You should be drinking half your body weight in ounces of water per day. For example, if you weigh 200 pounds, you should be drinking 100 ounces of water, but that's just a baseline.

>> **Ditch the coffee and alcohol.** If you're addicted to your morning latte, then at least try to decrease your intake. Both caffeine and alcohol are diuretics, meaning they make you urinate more and can worsen the dehydration that often occurs as you transition to keto (as glucose and glycogen leave your body, they carry three to four times their weight in water with it). Try reducing your intake of both beverages as you'll be chasing after your own tail — and getting nowhere fast — if you continue with the double espressos or after-dinner cocktails during your transition.

>> **Don't be afraid to take a rain check.** If you have the keto flu, you're probably not going to feel like going anywhere. Don't be afraid to let friends and family know that you'll have to reschedule something for another time. Relaxation and rest are very important — don't underestimate them!

When we first started the keto journey, we were ready to go all in. We fasted for two days, drinking water often and walking around a local park for an hour and a half each day to burn up our excess glycogen stores. We thought, "Faster is always better, right?" Not so fast. When day three hit, just as we began to get excited about digging into our avocado and coconut oil stores, the keto flu hit — and it hit hard. To say we felt like we had been run over by a truck was an understatement. We found it difficult to get out of bed, not only from fatigue, but also because as soon as we tried, the room immediately would go in and out of focus. Nausea hit like a ton of bricks, and we spent a lot of time in the bathroom. Both blood and urine tests showed that we were fully in ketosis, but being chained to the toilet put a damper on our celebration.

The moral of the story is that while going full bore will get you to ketosis faster, it isn't necessarily the healthiest — or most sustainable — way to go. If you're planning on kicking off ketosis with an intermittent fast and you're physically prepared and able, then go for it. But learn from our mistakes: Stay well hydrated and add some electrolyte water or even a bit of bone broth to your hydration regimen. If you start noticing symptoms or begin feeling unwell, make sure to have your favorite electrolyte replacement within easy reach. If you get a nasty case of keto flu, you'll be happy that you took some time to prepare for the worst-case scenario.

Watching for Signs of Ketoacidosis

We've already mentioned the difference between ketoacidosis and ketosis. You *want* to be in ketosis, but you must steer clear of ketoacidosis. Ketoacidosis can lead to life-threatening complications — the excess ketones make your body too acidic and shut down normal function.

Luckily, ketoacidosis is extremely rare when you transition to the keto diet. It primarily happens to people with type 1 diabetes, who tend to have high levels of blood glucose at the same time as high ketone levels. Because the natural biological process of transitioning to ketosis is to burn through all your glucose first, this almost never happens to someone who doesn't have a significant preexisting condition.

Less commonly, ketoacidosis is triggered by excessive exercise, starvation, severe alcohol abuse, or a severe illness. Even with these events, this condition occurs more commonly in a person who already has type 1 diabetes. Apart from being diabetic, research shows that women who start keto during pregnancy or when breastfeeding may also be at risk for ketoacidosis.

WARNING

Here are some signs that your symptoms are ketoacidosis and not just keto flu:

>> Excessive nausea and vomiting so much that you can't keep anything down

>> Urinating much more frequently throughout the day

>> Difficulty breathing or being unable to catch your breath

>> Extreme fatigue (to the point of being unable to get out of bed)

>> Fainting or "blacking out"

Ketoacidosis usually happens very suddenly — within a day — while keto flu usually takes a few days to show up.

You can test your ketones using urine test strips or checking blood levels. However, blood ketone levels will be more accurate than urine during your transition. That's because as your body begins to make more ketones, it may not be quite ready to use them efficiently, allowing the excess ketones to spill into your urine, artificially increasing the amount in your urine compared to the amount in your blood. As you get deeper into ketosis over the first few weeks, your urine ketone levels will drop as your body uses the available ketones more efficiently. Also, dehydration will spike your urine ketone levels compared to being hydrated. However, if your urine ketone levels are elevated and you have severe symptoms, you may be in ketoacidosis.

WARNING

If your ketone levels are in the range of ketoacidosis and you have significant symptoms, you should seek medical treatment immediately. Ketoacidosis is extremely rare when transitioning to keto. However, if your symptoms are extreme or you have a higher chance of having ketoacidosis due to a medical condition, don't wait to get medical help.

Addressing More Specific Side Effects

Keto flu is the main concern most people have as they transition to a keto lifestyle, but several other hiccups can occur at any point during your keto journey. Many of these issues will resolve with a little insight and awareness of the signs from your body. In this section, we break down common problems that you may encounter and how to fight them.

Cramps

Cramps are often the result of mineral imbalances, most commonly magnesium and potassium. When you're in ketosis, you'll lose more water from your body and, with it, electrolytes. Make sure you replace these regularly. The recommended daily allowances (RDAs) are:

>> **Magnesium:** 400 to 420 milligrams per day for men, 310 to 320 milligrams per day for women

>> **Potassium:** 4.7 grams per day for both men and women

It's best to get your minerals and electrolytes from whole foods, where they're usually in the right ratios to improve absorption. Both 1 ounce of almonds and ½ cup of spinach provide about 80 milligrams of magnesium per serving. On the other hand, 1 cup of avocado provides a whopping 700 milligrams of potassium, while a 3-ounce portion of chicken, beef, or salmon provides about 300 milligrams of this necessary nutrient. You definitely don't need a banana to fulfill your potassium requirements!

Other great remedies for muscle cramps include Epsom salt baths, a full body massage, and heat therapy.

Constipation

If you're dealing with constipation on the keto diet, know that you're not alone. Many people have experienced problems in this area even without going keto. Nearly one in five Americans have issues related to constipation, and things only worsen as we get older.

Constipation means different things for different people:

>> Difficulty or pain with passing bowel movements because they're hard or dry

>> Bowel movements that occur fewer than three times a week

Some people may go for five days or more without a bowel movement — ouch!

Although constipation is not unique to keto, as you transition, you lose a lot of your body water. This water was formerly attached to your carbohydrate stores and exits the body as you burn through glucose during the transition to ketosis. The key during this period is staying hydrated.

Also, many people aren't as familiar with keto-friendly sources of fiber and are likely to lose out on fiber-rich foods during this time. Yet, there are many options to decrease constipation as you transition, like fiber-filled nuts, fermented foods, and medium-chain triglyceride (MCT) oils. Your goal should be to eat about 25 to 30 grams of fiber (free carbs) a day.

TIP

Here are our top three tips to help improve constipation:

>> **Drink water.** Make sure you aren't dehydrated — this is one of the most common reasons for constipation. Water lubricates your intestines, allowing food to move smoothly through your system. Drinking the recommended amount of water makes you more regular and much less likely to have painful bowel movements. If it's been a few days, sip hot water on an empty stomach. This can help jumpstart your digestive system.

>> **Exercise.** Ever notice how the urge to go to the bathroom sometimes occurs just when you're in the middle of a workout? It's not your imagination: Exercise helps to improve flow to your gut, making you more receptive to having a bowel movement. Use this to your advantage if you're backed up!

>> **Put MCT in your coffee.** The memes on coffee mugs and T-shirts are true: Coffee can help bring on a much-needed trip to the bathroom. Although this shouldn't be your regular fallback option, it does work in a pinch. Adding MCT helps: It not only pushes you further into ketosis, but it also helps lubricate the gastrointestinal (GI) tract, allowing things to pass more smoothly. You can use coconut oil if you're out of MCT.

An oft-ignored fact is the physical position you use when having a bowel movement. Most people are pretty used to the porcelain throne, but the truth is that it may be worsening your constipation. You may have heard of the Squatty Potty (www.squattypotty.com) and wondered if there was anything to it. The idea is that if you raise your legs and lean forward, your body is at a better angle to facilitate the poop chute. Several scientific studies have confirmed this to be the case. So, if constipation is an issue, you can order a Squatty Potty online or simply put a little stool under your feet and lean forward at a 45-degree angle. Happy pooping!

TIP

There are many over-the-counter options to kick-start your digestive system if you're in a bind, but it's best to have a routine set up that includes hydration, fiber, and exercise to keep you regular and off of potentially habit-forming laxatives.

Diarrhea

Surprisingly, the opposite end of the spectrum, diarrhea, can show up during ketosis as well. It can rear its ugly head as you kick-start keto, just as it can any time you make a significant change in your eating habits. Generally, if diarrhea happens during your transition, it may be part of the keto flu, which you'll want to tackle from all sides. It'll improve as the flu resolves.

Diarrhea can also happen when you're deep into ketosis, especially when you add certain foods into your diet.

Two easy-to-fix reasons for keto-related diarrhea are

>> **Excess sugar alcohol sweeteners:** Erythritol, more so than xylitol, can lead to both stomach upset and diarrhea. This is highly variable as some people are more sensitive to sugar alcohols than others. If you notice more diarrhea after eating keto sweets, consider changing your sweetener to stevia or just reduce the amounts of keto treats you consume.

>> **MCT oil:** In the preceding section, we mention that MCT oil can help with a constipation issue, so it's not too surprising to find out that it can also push you too far in the opposite direction and lead to diarrhea. Some people who supplement with MCT oil to get into ketosis faster (and stay there) may notice this symptom. If this happens to you, reduce your intake of MCT oils (and coconut oil) for a while and slowly add them back in as your body learns to tolerate higher levels.

Another reason that diarrhea can happen is the significant increase in fats that you're consuming. If you've been eating a low-fat diet, your body won't be used to seeing and digesting the amount of fat you're now consuming. It takes time for your body to ramp up to handle all the fat-burning enzymes required to digest a 75 percent fat-based diet. Be patient and give your body time to take on this challenge.

If you're one of the approximately 300,000 Americans who've had your gallbladder removed, diarrhea on the keto diet may be even more of a problem. Your gallbladder stores much of your fat-burning enzymes as bile (see "Gallstones," later in this chapter). Some people — with or without a gallbladder — may not have enough of the enzymes necessary to digest and absorb the foods that they consume, leading to diarrhea. A digestive enzyme may be useful in these cases. Also, many people have low levels of stomach acid, which prevents them from being able to digest food as efficiently. Acid is one of the early tools you use to digest food and signals the pancreas to make digestive enzymes, which facilitate the process. If you have a lot of problems with heartburn, you may have low stomach acid levels.

To combat these issues, you'll want to choose an enzyme that has *lipase* (the main fat-digesting enzyme). Try adding a hydrochloric acid supplement to help boost your stomach acid levels as well. Be aware that medicines that treat heartburn tend to decrease the acid in your stomach; they may provide temporary heartburn relief, but they can also decrease your ability to digest food over the long term.

TIP

Although less common than constipation, keto can cause diarrhea. Common culprits are sugar alcohols, MCT oil, and increasing your fat intake too quickly.

Heart palpitations

Heart palpitations, or the feeling that your heart is beating way too hard or fast, can happen, especially during your transition to keto. Sometimes you feel like your heart skips a beat or is feathery. Although this sensation can provoke anxiety, do your best to stay calm because anxiety only makes the symptoms worse.

Heart palpitations during this period can be a result of the following:

>> Low blood sugar levels

>> Dehydration

>> Electrolyte abnormalities

TIP

If you notice palpitations as you transition, sit down and rest. Try drinking electrolyte water or broth to see if that helps. If you're concerned that your blood sugar levels are too low, this is a rare time that it's okay to eat a small amount of simple carbs. Options include a teaspoon of honey or maple syrup or a tablespoon of fruit juice.

Keto breath

If a friend mentions that your breath is beginning to stink during your transition, take it as a compliment — it might just mean you're in ketosis! Keto breath is often described as a "fruity breath," but our experience was more of a funny, almost metallic taste in the mouth and a fuzzy feeling to the tongue.

However it manifests for you, the culprit is one of the three ketones you'll encounter in your journey — acetone. If you or someone else notices this change to your breath, it means that you're producing acetone and more than likely the other two ketones. Bad breath usually isn't a cause for celebration, but know that you're moving into ketosis and your hard work is paying off. The good news is that keto breath is transitional and won't last long.

TIP

Don't be discouraged, keto breath should only last about a week or so. Here are our top four ways to minimize keto breath when it does occur:

>> Drink, drink, and drink more water.

>> Chew on mint leaves.

>> Pop a piece of sugar-free (xylitol) gum.

>> Chew on cinnamon bark.

WARNING

If keto breath lasts longer than a week or so, you may be eating too much protein. Remember that keto is a "moderate" protein diet. If your macros are off, the excess can break down into ammonia, another noxious-smelling substance that can make loved ones beg you to pop a breath mint.

Reduced strength or endurance

The transition to ketosis can be a trying time, sapping you of all your energy and making you feel as weak as a newborn. The reason is simple: Your body isn't used to ketosis and is still trying to run off of glycolysis, but you've stopped feeding it carbs. After you get into the swing of things, your body will quickly replace all its energy needs from fat, and you'll actually experience a more stable and consistent state of energy than you ever have before.

REMEMBER

In the meantime, however, take it easy and give yourself permission to rest. If this means sleeping nine or more hours a night for a few days, go with it — your body is telling you what it needs.

The eventual trade–off will be increased energy, mental focus, and vitality. Most people on keto find improved endurance, as well as an increased desire to move their bodies. As we've mentioned, multiple studies show that athletes who stick to a keto lifestyle have increased endurance and performance compared to athletes who eat more carbs. Keto also helps to improve learning and memory in people with Alzheimer's disease and other forms of dementia. The diet has a track record of improving your performance in a variety of areas over the long term.

TIP

If it's been more than a few weeks since you've transitioned and you're feeling tired and weak, it's time to problem–solve. Here are some common reasons for continued lethargy during ketosis:

>> **Dehydration:** Remember that on keto, you lose more water than on a carbohydrate-heavy diet. If you're always tired, make sure you're drinking enough fluids.

>> **Imbalance in electrolytes:** As you lose water, you lose salt. Keep up with your electrolytes, and you'll likely see an improvement in energy.

>> **Nutritional deficit:** You may default to eating the same two or three meals that you know are keto-friendly. Unfortunately, although these meals may fit in with the macros, you may be missing some of the vital micronutrients. If you have a vitamin deficiency, it often will show up as pervasive fatigue that is difficult to treat. Get creative and try new keto-friendly foods that are rich in vitamins and minerals. If all else fails, taking a good multivitamin may be helpful.

>> **Eating too few calories:** It can be hard to eat as many calories as you need on the keto diet because you'll find that you aren't as hungry. Also, because your food is so nutrient-dense, you'll be eating a lot less than you used to. If you're trying to lose weight fast, don't slash calories too quickly. On keto, your carb cravings tend to disappear, so it's surprisingly easy to drop your total daily calories. Whichever food lifestyle you follow, if you eat too few calories based on your activity level, you'll end up feeling weak and lackluster.

Hair loss

The ketogenic diet should not, in and of itself, cause hair loss. If you suddenly notice more hair clogging the sink after transitioning to keto, it's likely a period of transition that happens as you make a substantial lifestyle change. Keto can be extremely beneficial for your health, but any sudden and drastic change to your daily routine can affect hair growth.

Here are four common reasons keto is associated with sudden hair loss:

>> Eating or drinking too few calories per day

>> Nutritional deficiency (not getting enough vitamins and minerals)

>> Not meeting your protein requirements

>> High levels of stress

Some of these triggers are similar to the ones that lead to extreme fatigue. Your body is very practical. If it doesn't get the right level of nutrients it needs, it will use whatever energy is available to nourish vital organs (like your heart), and secondary areas (like your hair and nails) will suffer the consequences. Because there isn't much energy left to go around if you're eating too little, you'll feel tired, so don't go to CrossFit and make the energy deficit even worse.

If you're eating too few calories, this may be the cause of your hair loss. Even if you want to lose weight, you shouldn't cut more than about 500 calories a day. Use the Mifflin–St. Jeor equation (see Chapter 7) to determine how many calories you should be eating. Adding an extra avocado or some coconut oil to your meal are great ways to add nutrient-dense calories quickly.

Also, check out your protein intake and make sure it's moderate. Your goal should be about 20 percent of your total intake or 0.36 to 0.45 gram of protein per pound of body weight (or more if you're very active). Adding some nuts to your diet or eating a hard-boiled egg on the go is a quick, easy, and keto-friendly way to increase your protein.

If you're still losing hair, make sure you're including these hair-thickening nutrients in your daily diet:

>> **Biotin:** Biotin, one of the B vitamins, is important for energy metabolism and is often a component of hair and nail multivitamins because it strengthens and thickens both of these areas. Some studies suggest that very low-carb diets are associated with a deficiency in biotin. Make sure to supplement by eating biotin-rich foods like egg yolks, avocados, and salmon. You should aim for at least 30 milligrams of biotin per day.

>> **Methylsulfonylmethane (MSM):** This is a nutrient that helps to maintain the structure in the body, including the skin, nails, and hair. It's also a common component of supplements for joint health because it helps to decrease inflammation. You can naturally find MSM in many animal foods like raw milk, as well as vegetables like leafy greens and tomatoes. Choose uncooked versions to get the most MSM; heat may decrease the amount of the nutrient.

>> **Zinc:** This essential mineral is vital for a host of body processes, including healthy skin and thyroid function. If you have low levels of zinc, you put yourself at risk for thyroid disease, which is a prevalent cause of hair loss. You'll also exacerbate any skin conditions you may already have. To combat this, there are several keto-friendly zinc sources like grass-fed beef, chicken, and cacao powder.

>> **Collagen:** You've probably seen a combination of collagen and MSM supplements for healthy joints. Collagen is a major component of the cells that stimulate your hair to grow, helps prevent damage to your hair follicles, and may even reduce graying. We tend to stop making collagen as we age, so it's important to supplement this nutrient over time. A great way to add collagen to your diet is to sip on bone broth. You can also choose to add some vitamin C to your diet, which helps boost your natural production of collagen. Some keto-friendly vitamin C sources include brussels sprouts and bell peppers.

A quick word about stress: As you make any significant life change, stress is likely to happen. Whether it's breaking up with your favorite high-carb foods, talking with housemates or friends about your decision to go keto, or the toll of the keto flu, stress can show up as hair loss. When you're stressed, your body speeds up the life cycle of each individual hair, which naturally culminates in hair falling out. This, of course, slows down when stress levels drop. For many people on the keto diet, this stressed hair cycle can last up to a few months, but it's primarily due to stress rather than ketosis.

WARNING

Rarely, hair loss can be a sign of a deeper underlying illness. The stress from going through keto can unmask an underlying health condition like thyroid disease or anemia, which can also cause hair loss. If you're experiencing other symptoms that indicate something deeper is at play, talk with your doctor to find out what's going on.

High cholesterol

Many people may try to suggest that keto is unhealthy, not only because of the high-fat content, but also because of the amount of cholesterol you'll naturally eat. We've totally debunked this myth by showing that not only does fat not make you fat, but the cholesterol (you eat) does not result in bad cholesterol levels. It's more likely that donuts and low-fat muffins are worsening your cholesterol levels than the possibility of eggs and grass-fed beef doing so. This may be hard for many people to wrap their minds around, but increasing amounts of scientific evidence show this to be true.

As we mention in Chapter 4, cholesterol levels are typically broken down into high-density lipoprotein (HDL, the "good" kind) and low-density lipoprotein (LDL, the "bad" kind), but the story is a little more complicated than that. Everyone agrees that HDL is associated with a lower risk for heart disease, but new information about LDL is complicating simplistic views of cholesterol.

It's essential to break down LDL and understand that it isn't universally "bad." LDL comes in several forms:

>> Small, dense LDL is the real bad guy. This is the cholesterol that is associated with heart disease, obesity, and stroke.

>> Large, buoyant LDL is much less inflammatory and is not closely correlated to any of these complications.

>> Intermediate LDL is slightly smaller than the large, buoyant LDL and acts very similar to it.

As you can see, if you have high LDL, it really makes a difference if you have more of the small, dense LDL versus the large or intermediate LDL, which isn't as bad. Unfortunately, this difference isn't appreciated when you get your cholesterol levels checked. The tests that differentiate types of LDL are relatively expensive and not widely available, so your doctor likely isn't testing to look for these subtle differences.

Here is a quick overview of how certain types of foods affect your cholesterol test levels:

>> Fats (monounsaturated fatty acids [MUFAs], omega-3s, and saturated fats like MCT oils) increase HDL, while carbs decrease them.

>> MCT oils (including coconut oil) decrease triglyceride levels. Triglycerides are another component of your annual cholesterol check; they represent free-flowing fat in your bloodstream and increase your risk of heart disease.

>> Consuming high glycemic-index foods (simple carbs) increases overall blood cholesterol more than eating foods high in cholesterol.

>> Saturated fat raises the large, buoyant kind of LDL, while simple carbs increase the small, dense LDL.

Overall, a very low-carbohydrate diet, like keto, increases large, buoyant LDL, increases HDL, and decreases triglycerides. The keto diet improves all areas of blood cholesterol, even if people often overlook its subtle benefits at first glance.

Overall, keto can be more heart-healthy than eating a standard American diet, where carbohydrates make up about 50 percent to 55 percent of daily intake and too many of the calories come from simple carbs.

REMEMBER

Fat does not make you fat, and keto doesn't worsen your cholesterol levels. On the other hand, eating too many carbs can do both.

Gallstones

You may have heard that eating fat increases your chance of getting gallstones. The gallbladder is a little organ tucked underneath your liver that stores — but does not make — bile. *Bile* is a greenish liquid that helps digest the fat in your food and is released when you eat a meal high in fats. Your pancreas makes most of the fat-digesting enzymes you need and transfers it to the gallbladder to be stored. The prevailing logic is that people who eat a lot of fat overtax their gallbladders, which increases their chance of forming *gallstones* (little calcified balls that may block the flow of bile over time). Gallstones can lead to intense pain in the right side of your belly that is often treated with surgery to remove the organ.

Many of the studies showing an increase in gallstones with keto diet have looked at children using keto to treat epilepsy. The other group at increased risk are people who cut their daily calories substantially and eat very low-fat diets. A study of 22 overweight people who were on very low-calorie diets (only about 500 calories a day) and ate minimal amounts of fat were more likely to get gallstones than people who were on the same low-calorie regimen but ate higher percentages of fat. In the study, the difference between the two groups' diets was about 3 grams of fat versus 12 grams of fat.

The scientists concluded that eating fat actually helps to flush out the gallbladder rather than overtax it. As you can imagine, the people eating very little fat had a stagnant pool of bile that, over time, began to calcify and form stones. The big caveat is that if you already have a gallstone, eating fat can help push it out, but if it gets stuck on the way, you may end up with intense gallbladder pain. So, if you already have gallstones and start the keto diet, you may experience pain as the gallstones try to work their way out of your system. The good news is that many people can pass their gallstones on their own with some time.

Another important question that comes up for some people when starting the keto diet is whether it's possible to go keto if you've already had your gallbladder removed. After all, the gallbladder plays a crucial role in helping you digest the nutrient-rich fat found in keto foods. Never fear: Because the gallbladder only *stores* the bile, your pancreas will be able to gear up and make the critical digestive enzymes to help you digest your food.

WARNING

If you've just had your gallbladder removed, this process may be a little slow because the pancreas doesn't have an easy storage house for the enzymes. Over time, however, your body will get used to storing bile without the gallbladder, and you'll likely be able to increase your daily fat intake quite a bit. It's vital, however, that you take your time, so in this situation, it's best to slowly ease into keto instead of trying to transition within a day or two.

Indigestion

Indigestion, or heartburn, is a common problem that many Americans face. It's so common that formerly prescription-strength heartburn medications like Nexium and Prevacid are now available over the counter at your local drugstore. Most Americans are not on the keto diet, so it's hard to blame keto for causing this issue. That being said, indigestion can be caused by a sudden change in your eating habits (keto or otherwise). Another common cause is reflux disease, where the acid from the stomach moves back into your esophagus, burning it.

Heartburn is worsened by excessive coffee, cigarettes, and alcohol. If you're having a lot of indigestion, and commonly use any of these, consider cutting back. Also, people with thyroid disorders, who use excessive over-the-counter antacids, prescription heartburn medicines, or pain medications (like ibuprofen and aspirin) are at risk.

TIP

You can use three comprehensive strategies to help combat indigestion:

» **Cut out irritants.** Common irritants are cigarettes, coffee, and alcohol. Consider cutting out all dairy (except butter and ghee) for two or three days and see if this helps. Many people have trouble digesting the lactose in dairy products; for these folks, lactose is often a cause of indigestion and bloating. Also, "acidic" foods like tomatoes can worsen your indigestion.

Try keeping a food diary to see if certain foods trigger indigestion for you. If you identify any, remove them from your diet for relief.

» **Slow down and chew your food.** Really. Chewing and mixing food with your saliva is the first — and most important — step in digestion. If you gulp food down, your stomach must do extra work to break it down, which can lead to the telltale signs of heartburn. Well-digested food means less indigestion. This "mindful" eating also helps you recognize the early signs of satiety, so you can stop eating when your body tells you that you're done.

>> **Supplement.** An unhealthy gut will affect all aspects of your digestion and can worsen indigestion. If your gut bacteria are unhappy, you'll end up with bloating, flatulence, and indigestion. Combat this by eating fermented foods like sauerkraut and drinking apple cider vinegar to replenish your good gut bacteria. If you don't enjoy fermented foods, invest in a good daily probiotic for gut health. Make sure it has adequate levels of both *Bifidobacterium* and *Lactobacillus,* the most important bacteria for your digestive system. Generally speaking, there should be at least 1 billion colony forming units (CFUs) in any probiotic you take.

TIP

If you're having a particularly difficult time and you need a quick remedy, we've found that adding a teaspoon of baking soda and a squeeze of lime to a full glass of water can do the trick. This combination decreases both the heartburn and the gas associated with indigestion. Remember to drink water throughout the day — it will help to reduce stomach acid to proper levels, so it's a great way to decrease the symptoms of heartburn.

The heartburn associated with keto may worsen during your transition, but it should slowly settle as you get into the routine of keto. Some people notice that, over the long term, going keto may actually improve their symptoms of indigestion. Their improvement happens because grain — and especially gluten-containing carbs — are a common trigger for indigestion for many people.

Rashes

When we first started the keto diet, Vicky noticed an intensely red and itchy rash that suddenly showed up on her neck, back, chest, and belly. This was alarming because we'd just watched a documentary on the "flesh-eating bacteria" and were terrified that this was somehow the cause of the severe rash. That led to an Internet search, which only added fuel to our already overexcited imaginations. If this is what you were thinking, don't worry — you didn't pick up a deadly bacterium, and you will survive to see another day.

The *keto rash* is not unique to keto, yet multiple scientific reports show that people transitioning onto keto are more likely to develop a rash. It also happens to people who drastically change their diets in other ways; for example, new vegans or people going on an intense weight loss diet can also get a rash.

Why some people get rashes is unclear, but it does have a specific name: *prurigo pigmentosa. Prurigo* refers to the intense itching, while *pigmentosa* refers to the dark patches that are often left behind after the rash disappears. The keto rash more commonly happens to people with diabetes who begin eating a very low-carb diet. Interestingly, it also seems to be more common in people of Japanese descent — the vast majority of studies of people dealing with the rash were done in Japan.

The appearance of the rash can be quite dramatic, and it can even become scaly over time. Many people notice that the outbreak will resolve itself, but it can also return without warning. If it keeps recurring, you're more likely to get dark patches that don't go away between episodes. Some researchers think keto rash is an allergic reaction to certain foods, which only becomes apparent when you drastically change your diet and are exposed to these foods. The rash could also be related to nutrition deficits because you've cut the variety of foods you eat on keto. Finally, it may be that ketones your body releases when you sweat are irritating and inflaming your skin, causing the telltale rash over your body.

Here are a few ways to deal with keto rash:

» **Minimize the amount you sweat.** Try to keep cool if it's summertime, and take a break from any intense exercise. Because the ketones you sweat out may be leading to the rash, staying away from the gym for a while may help stop the irritation and give you relief from constant itching.

» **Supplement.** Keto rash, like many other rashes, is often caused by increasing inflammation in your skin. Transitioning to keto without eating a variety of whole foods can lead to deficiencies in many of the nutrients that are important for skin health, including zinc, vitamin C, and B vitamins. If you're transitioning and you aren't getting enough of these nutrients, diversify the types of foods you eat and consider taking a balanced daily multivitamin.

» **Cut out food allergies.** If you suddenly start eating new foods that weren't typical for you before starting the keto diet, this may be causing an allergic reaction. Common keto foods that many people are allergic to are eggs, nuts, seafood, and dairy. Try eliminating these foods from your diet to see if it helps to stop the spread of keto rash.

» **Fight inflammation.** Consume anti-inflammatory and antioxidant foods or supplements that contain omega-3 fatty acids and probiotics. The probiotics are important because some researchers believe that an unhealthy gut affects every part of your body. This includes your skin and can show up as angry and irritated keto rash.

The keto rash can go away on its own, but it may take a few months. It's hard to deal with intense itchiness for that long, so try some of these options to attack the problem. Also, remember that it can come back again — in some studies, the back and forth lasted for years!

TIP

If your keto rash is severe and won't go away despite trying all these home remedies, it may be time to make an appointment with your doctor. He or she may be able to prescribe an antibiotic to help treat the rash.

A final option you can consider is to increase your carb intake. In several studies, going off the keto diet and reversing ketosis treated the condition and the keto rash went away. All is not lost: You don't have to go back to the standard high-carb diet — many people came out of ketosis but still maintained a relatively low-carb diet in the range of 100 to 150 grams of carbs per day. Some people slowly increase their carbs while in ketosis and may even find a sweet spot that allows them to increase their carbs without being completely kicked out of ketosis. Even if the rash doesn't resolve before you get out of ketosis, you can slowly work your way back into ketosis by gradually decreasing your carb intake over time.

REMEMBER

The keto rash is rare. Most people on keto don't get it, so don't let this be a deterrent to going keto.

Chapter **11**

Alleviating Any Social Pressure

Whenever you take the first step toward committing to a significant life change, a feeling of resistance is likely to rear its ugly head. Think back to a time when you decided to do something that, at first, you may not have entirely believed you could accomplish. Whether it was completing your first marathon or pledging to save a portion of your paycheck every month, you likely came across a few hurdles and seriously considered quitting a few times. That's the way things go when you decide to reach for your goals — the outcome is always worth it, but it won't always be smooth sailing.

Resistance can come from within yourself, or it can be externally placed on you by people whose opinions you trust and respect. Sometimes, this resistance can feel like a brick wall that you just can't push through, no matter how many times you try. With time, we're better equipped to differentiate our needs from our wants and realize that our goals may not always fall in line with public opinion or even the approval of our loved ones.

When you've thoroughly researched keto, determined that it's the right choice for you, and started the journey, you may have to let go of others' opinions of what you should or shouldn't eat. Just as important, you'll have to let go of fears that keto is not possible for you or that you don't deserve to put your health first. Don't let your desire for approval or your familiarity with the status quo deter you from reaching your goal.

In this chapter, we give you some useful reminders and tips on how to stop the naysayers from derailing your keto journey.

Staying Focused

Unfortunately, the first naysayer most of us need to deal with is the one that stares back at us from the mirror each morning. Self-doubt can come in the form of that nagging little voice in your head that tells you keto is impossible, even though you haven't begun to try and deep down you know you're strong enough to make it happen. Going against decades of nutritional tradition can be difficult. Many people who are starting the keto journey may balk at the thought of eating so much fat or ditching "healthy whole grains." Over time, we've internalized the belief that "low fat is best," despite our bodies telling us otherwise and our waist-lines continuously expanding.

Take time to acknowledge this little voice and understand that it's merely a seed of doubt and doesn't have to define your journey. Whenever you go against conventional wisdom, you may encounter intense resistance to the road less traveled. That's a sign of growth and that you're empowering yourself to reach for your personal goals. The best way to squelch this fear is to conduct research and reassure yourself that this is indeed the best choice for you. Make a commitment to go keto and see the benefits for yourself.

Here are some basic first steps to set yourself up for success:

>> **Eliminate high-carb foods from your kitchen.** Give these foods to a friend who isn't on keto or donate them to a local food shelter, so they don't go to waste.

>> **Stock up on keto-friendly whole foods.** Stay away from the aisles of grocery stores where all the high-carb junk can be found. Instead, focus on the well-stocked meat and dairy sections, as well as whole, nutritious, low-carb veggies. Get adventurous and go to local ethnic grocery stores and try keto-friendly foods you may have never tried before. Check out Middle Eastern grocers for *labneh,* a soft, creamy cheese that's a great option for breakfast, or go to an Italian grocer to stock up on antipasti favorites like cured meats, hard cheeses, and a variety of low-carb veggies. Take a look at Chapter 5 to see the best ingredients to get, and look at Part 5 of this book to come up with food lists.

>> **Get support from a good friend or loved one who can be a shoulder to lean on if you go through the keto flu.** If you have a friend who is starting keto at the same time, that's best, but make sure it's a friend whom you feel comfortable sharing your triumphs and failures with and who will be there to

support you through the hard times. A great friend will remind you of your goals and encourage you to let go of the donut when your resolve weakens.

» **Clearly identify your reasons for making the change to keto.** Whether you want to treat diabetes and get rid of blood sugar medications, or you're tired of constant fatigue and low energy, make sure you identify all the reasons for keto so you can hold on to them throughout your journey and celebrate reaching your goals.

TIP

This last point isn't just an abstract exercise: You should write down your goals and post them where you can see them every day. For example, write down what you'll accomplish when you're off all your blood sugar medications or put a collage of yourself at your ideal weight relaxing on a beach. Place this picture or motivational statement on your fridge or your bathroom mirror for the best effect. We know of someone who recorded a list of all the reasons she was going keto and how she hoped it would improve her life and turned the recording into her daily alarm. Be creative and do what works for you. When you step in with this motivation and set up tools to keep your momentum going, you're much more likely to go all the way on your journey.

REMEMBER

Don't get too stuck on a timeline for completely transitioning to a keto lifestyle. You may have heard that if you stick with something for 21 days, it becomes an automatic habit, but that's just a commonly held myth. The reality is that creating a habit is much more variable; some people can easily stick to a lifestyle change after only three weeks, but others can try for more than eight months before the shift feels automatic. Be kind to yourself as you go on the keto journey, realizing it's a marathon, not a sprint. More important, don't judge your progress by comparing it to anyone else's, or it'll just set you up for disappointment. Others may move faster or slower than you; their plateaus may come before or after yours. This journey is completely customized to you, and you shouldn't measure your success by how others are doing.

In psychology, there are six steps to making a permanent life change (called the *Transtheoretical Model*):

» **Precontemplation:** You have a vague idea that you want to make a change in your life, but you don't yet have enough motivation to try it; perhaps you think it'll be too difficult. This is you if you've heard about keto and you're aware of its benefits, but you don't feel you have any reason to make such a drastic change in your life and you're skeptical of letting go of your cereal and low-fat bagel habit. It's tough to make a change if you're in this stage.

» **Contemplation:** You're seriously thinking about making a change and you want to learn more about what it would take. You may not be ready to jump headfirst, but you're open to the benefits of making a change. Perhaps you know a little bit about keto and you're sure that you want to improve your health, but you aren't certain how to make the change. This book is a great low-stress way to delve a bit deeper and reinforce all the fantastic benefits that keto has to offer.

» **Preparation:** You're willing and wanting to move forward. You know you want to go keto, but you still need some guidance and motivation to get started. Perhaps you've looked up some recipes, or you're aware of the benefits of keto for your health and energy, but you need to take a serious look at making a plan for your journey. Chapters 5 and 6 are excellent tools to have in your back pocket so you have a detailed plan of what foods you should be stocking up on. It's also a great idea to seek out keto support groups online or check out some of the keto resources in Chapter 23 for motivation.

» **Action:** You're ready to jump in. You've got your plan set up, you're clear on why you're going keto, and you've got your motivation written on your fridge. It's critical during this stage that you have a personal supporter who will help you stay motivated when you're going through the keto flu or if you're headed to a work party where there will be tons of high-carb treats. This is where all your preparation pays off. This phase is not static — there may be ups and downs. Remember that creating the feeling that things are automatic could take weeks or months.

» **Maintenance:** Things are beginning to get intuitive. You start your day off with a mini baked quiche or you do intermittent fasting without giving it a second thought. You've got your alternative keto sides ready to go at your favorite restaurant, and you know how keto "works" in your life. You've seen the benefits in your life, and you're confident that keto can be a long-term lifestyle for you. However, at this stage, a substantial change — a significant breakup, a move across the country, or even a plateau in your weight loss — may make your journey seem rocky. It can seem even more frustrating if you slide back to old patterns during this stage, but remember: It's a journey and you can always start back up again. Your body doesn't lose the ability to get back into ketosis, and you'll still reap the same benefits when you go back to it. In fact, after you've gone through the fat adaptation process once, your body will transition into it much more efficiently on subsequent attempts.

» **Termination:** This is when everything is ingrained. Keto is simply part of your life — it's not something you consciously think about anymore. Even when you're surrounded by a bread basket, you have no desire to eat it. You understand the benefits of keto, and it's effortless. Be aware that it can take years to feel this level of comfort with a lifestyle change.

In the action stage, many people start off extremely motivated, ready to tackle any keto obstacle with gusto. But remember, during any transition, there are always a few hurdles to overcome. We call this the "quicksand" period, because almost everything seems like a trap trying to drag you away from your keto goal. Keto meals somehow seem boring, you're almost on empty on the motivation scale, or you're tired of explaining to one more person why you won't eat the rice or bread or potatoes.

For many people, this happens during the keto flu. The same thing happened to us because we went through a particularly rough bout of keto flu during our transition. Our symptoms were so severe that we could barely drag ourselves to work and, when we did, it was just to stare blankly at the computer screen and not get anything done. When you go out looking like that, people wonder why you're putting yourself through an extreme diet — and you may start to question it yourself. Justifying our decision got old pretty quickly, and to be honest, we thought about quitting a few times. Luckily, we had each other for support and had almost no carbs at home, so we made it through this rough patch. The key is recognizing that this is a normal part of the process of forming a healthy lifestyle, and it will get better over time.

This is an excellent time to let your imagination run free. Imagine how things will be if you get to the other side of this hump. Ask yourself how you'll feel having committed to keto for a full three months. Also, imagine what it would feel like to give up on keto and have to face starting over again with the possibility of reliving keto flu in a few weeks. Really make an effort to let both scenarios take hold of your imagination and allow yourself to feel the satisfaction, disappointment, or irritation associated with each scenario. This exercise really helps to build motivation during difficult times.

TIP

We found another great way to overcome the challenges of the action phase was to keep a keto diary. We started it on the first day we went keto, but you should feel free to start it at any point in your journey. We made a commitment to write in our journals every morning, recording everything from the struggles of keto flu to the triumph of one month strong on keto. Having a record of these milestones helped relieve frustration, as well as gave us hope when things seemed particularly difficult. Being reminded of the amazing changes we went through, including increased energy, vitality, and weight loss were incredibly motivating. As you see the results for yourself and keto becomes personal, you'll quiet that voice that wants to tell you to quit.

REMEMBER

You may be your own biggest critic. Take the time now to set yourself up for success by removing common obstacles that you inadvertently set up for yourself.

Letting Your Social Circle in on Your Journey

First, know that your (true) friends and family will want what's best for you and your health. If you're sure that starting the keto journey is the best thing for your overall well-being — and you've put in the preparation — the people in your life will likely come around to your way of thinking. If they don't, you'll need to be okay with their decision and realize you can't force others to change their minds. When you embrace this attitude, you'll find out if you can make things work with their tacit disapproval or if you'll need to take a step back from the relationship.

Find someone whose opinion you trust and respect; then get her involved in your decision to go keto. Whether it's a friend who's already made a healthy lifestyle change in his life or a loved one whom you respect and have looked up to since you were a child, choose wisely. Let her know why you've decided to go keto and use her as an ally to get through tough patches like keto flu or the "quicksand" period. Make sure the person you choose is easily accessible, either in person or by phone, for the times when the going gets tough.

If you're worried about letting your loved ones know that you're going keto, dig deep and try to figure out why this is the case. For example, you may fear that they'll judge you for making a change in your diet. Perhaps you're a little ashamed because it's your 15th "diet change" and you're worried that they won't believe this one will stick.

Whatever is true for you, come to terms with it and realize that your health and well-being are more important than any of these fears. Don't beat yourself up for having these fears — they're completely natural when you open yourself up to other people's opinions about you. This is being vulnerable, and it's a rare strength that often comes with more benefits than you realize. Telling your coworkers that you're going keto after they've seen you fail at your last five diets may leave you open to ridicule, but focus instead on the potential support you could get from coworkers who are looking for someone to be their support when they're struggling with the transition.

After you've worked through your concerns, it's time to get clear about your expectations. For example:

>> Do you want your significant other to start keto with you?

>> Do you want your housemate to stop buying potato chips and bread?

>> Do you want your family to accept your decision and try not to change your mind?

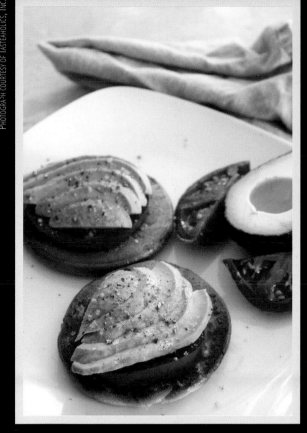

Avocado Cloud Toast (Chapter 14)

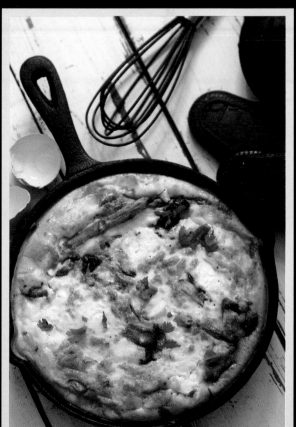

Goat Cheese Frittata (Chapter 14)

Lemon Kale Salad (Chapter 15)

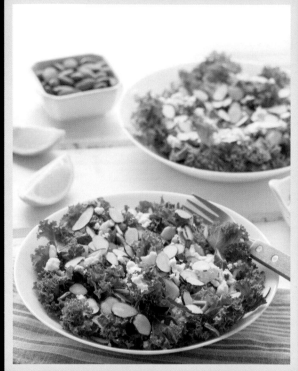

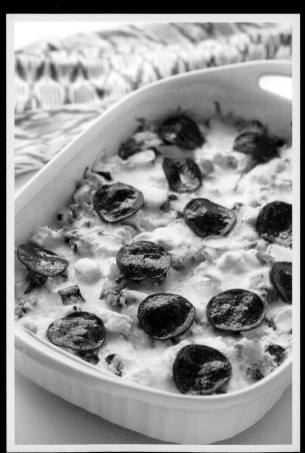

Chicken Pizza Casserole (Chapter 15)

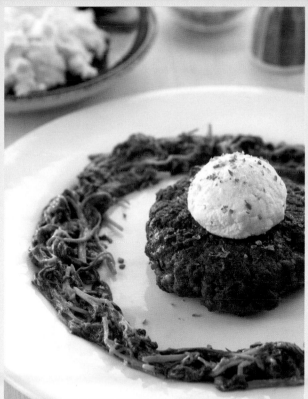

Mediterranean Lamb Burgers (Chapter 16)

Extra-Crispy Chicken Thighs (Chapter 16)

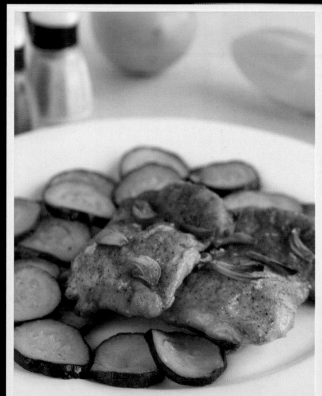

Cheesy Baked Asparagus (Chapter 17)

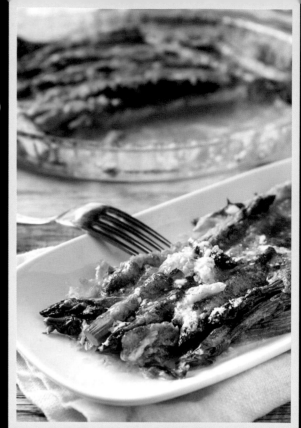

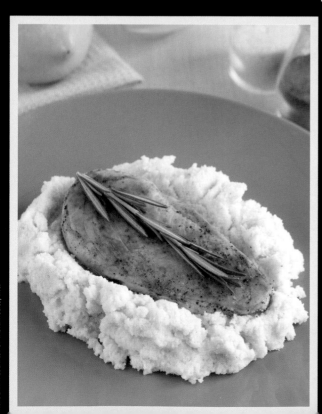

**Cauliflower Mash with Browned Butter
(Chapter 17) and Lemon Rosemary Chicken**

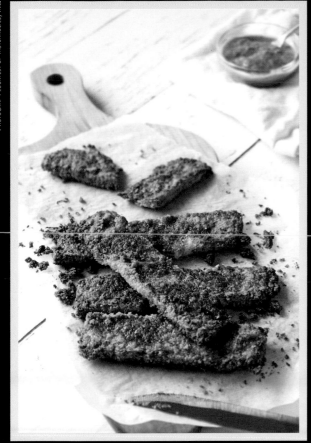

Pesto Bread Strips (Chapter 18)

Cheese Chips and Guacamole (Chapter 18)

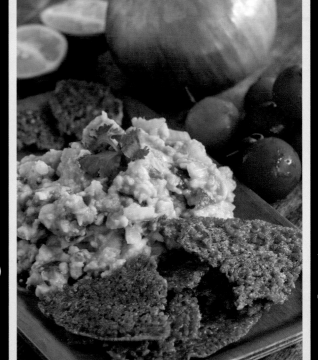

Butternut Squash Soup (Chapter 19)

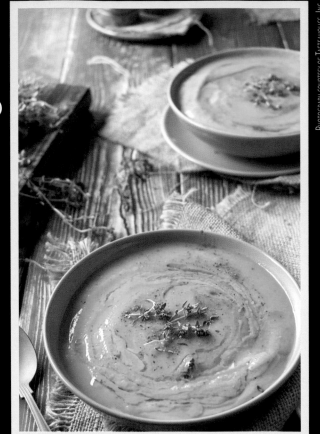

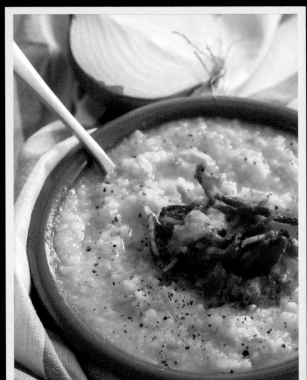

One-Pot Creamy Cauliflower Chowder (Chapter 19)

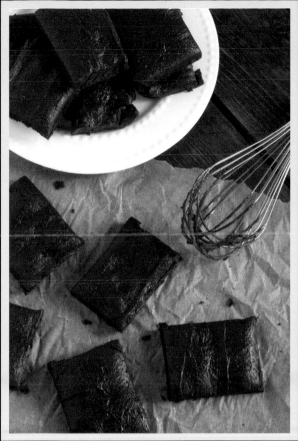

Almond Fudge Brownies (Chapter 20)

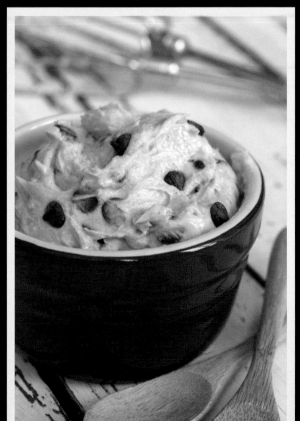

Creamy Cookie Dough Mousse (Chapter 20)

Avocado Chocolate Mousse (Chapter 20)

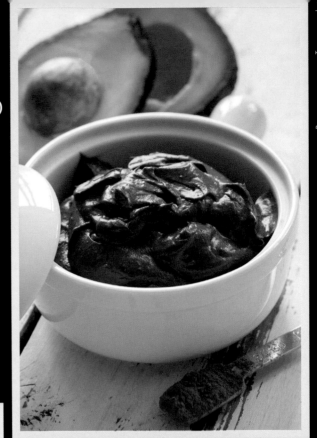

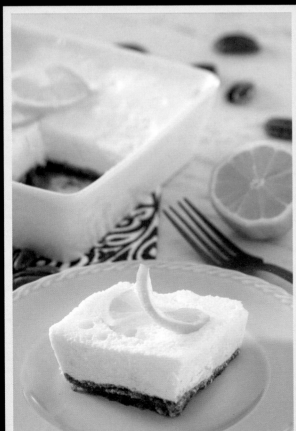

Lemon Jell-O Cake (Chapter 20)

All of these may happen, but some are much more likely than others. You'll need to figure out which ones are possible, as well as which are critical for your success in going keto.

Treat discussing keto with friends and family as you would treat speaking to them about any topic you're passionate about. There's no need to talk their ears off if they're uninterested, but let them know why you're excited about keto and that you're committed to it. Your family is unlikely to scoff at your plans for your career if you've been at it for the last few years; in the same way, you shouldn't have to deal with them being derisive about your eating habits if you're just as committed to that.

Be clear about what going keto means for your eating habits, especially if you get a home-cooked meal from your parents once a month or share the grocery bill with your housemate. You don't want it to be a shock when you stop paying for your share of the potato chips or when you tell your mom that, no, you won't be partaking in her famous sweet potato pie anymore. You'll need to have an open discussion before these things come to a head.

It's also important not to become a zealot or scoff at friends and family when they bring out their whole-grain granola or choose the sweet potato fries as the healthier snack. Going keto is not an excuse to become a judge of everyone else's dinner plate — that's the best way to make a lot of enemies very quickly. Just like anyone deciding to go keto, everyone else has the right to make his own food choices and nourish himself with the foods he feels are best for him.

REMEMBER

If you're hoping that others will join the keto journey with you, it's best to let go of that hope. You can't force others to make a permanent lifestyle change if they aren't willing to do it. The best you can hope for is that they'll see the benefits you gain and decide to make the change for themselves over time. Actions speak a lot louder than words.

TIP

Here are a few tips we found to be helpful in making the transition smoother with non-keto friends and family:

>> **Make your opinions clear and honest.** Let everyone know why keto is important to you — without lecturing on how carbs are the enemy. You may feel that way, but you won't convert anyone to keto by getting on your soapbox. Instead, let the changes in your health speak for you.

>> **Be consistent.** Don't "cheat" when you eat at your parents' house or when you go out to dinner with friends. When friends and family see you saying one thing and doing another, it undermines your commitment to keto and leaves them feeling skeptical about your decision.

» **Let friends or family know beforehand that you won't be eating any high-carb foods if you're invited to dinner.** It's best to do this before the event, instead of showing up and only drinking water the whole night. You may ultimately decide that you'll eat a small meal before going to a dinner party if there will be almost nothing you can eat or ask them if they wouldn't mind making sure that there are some keto options.

» **Bring one of your favorite keto foods to a potluck or offer to cook a keto meal with a loved one.** This is one of the quickest ways to get them onboard and show how diverse and satisfying a keto meal can be. When we were invited to a friend's potluck, we brought over the Creamy Cookie Dough Mousse (Chapter 20). No one could believe that it was essentially sugar-free, and everyone was clamoring for the recipe. It really opened up even the most sugar-addicted of our friends to the mind-set that keto is possible for everyone.

Be prepared for concerned looks and fears about your heart health and a lecture or two about all the ways a "bacon and cheese diet" will kill you. Take all this in stride and with the long view of educating your family and friends. There are a lot of misconceptions about the keto diet, and you're likely to hear it all when people know that you're going keto. Hearing the same concerns may get tiresome after a while, but remember that many of your friends were fed the same misinformation and that you, too, likely held many of the same misconceptions before you went keto. Let your concerned friends and family know that keto actually has a lot of scientific merit to it, which you're aware of and which has the backing of nutritionists, doctors, and researchers who take the time to understand it.

You may unintentionally become a keto ambassador. How much or how little education you want to provide to others is up to you. We found that the deeper we got into keto and the more research we read, the more we wanted to shout out all of its benefits to everyone who would listen. That's obviously one of the reasons we started the Tasteaholics website and wrote this book. However, that may not be the case for you — keto is intensely personal and private for some people. You can point your family and friends to good research (like this book!), or you can give a little spiel about the health benefits you've had on keto and clear up the misconception that you eat bacon 24/7. There is no need to try to force others to adopt your way of eating; your results will speak much more loudly than anything you say.

WARNING

We should point out that living with a housemate or someone else who is not onboard with keto can put a bit of a wrench in your transition. Cleaning out your pantry may be a little bit more challenging if your housemate has bags of cookies, potato chips, or other high-carb treats stored there that would cause a mini civil war if you gave them away without your housemate's consent. You'll need to have a frank conversation with your housemate and try to come up with a mutually beneficial agreement. Perhaps he'll want to go keto after you let him know about all its benefits!

TIP

If housemates aren't quite ready to go keto, here are some simple tricks to decrease temptations when off-limit foods are readily available:

>> **If you split the grocery bill, stop!** Tell your housemates that you'll have to start buying groceries separately because you won't be eating a lot of the high-carb foods that they'll want to buy. You'll probably find it easier to refrain from eating the potato chips if you didn't pay for them. This will stop any unhappiness that can arise from any of you because you're paying for foods you'd rather not eat.

>> **Divide the pantry shelves and fridge space.** Ask your housemates if they can put all their carbs in a specific area so that you can train yourself over time to ignore that space. For example, if you're short, ask them to put all the cookies and chips on the top shelf, where it will be harder for you to access them.

>> **Ask your housemates if they'd be okay with your writing the number of grams of carbs per serving on packaged food items in big red letters.** This is a great trick to dissuade you from biting into a chip or other goodie when your willpower gets a little weak.

Now's a good time to take the initiative and seek out others who are on the keto journey. You can plan on joining a Facebook group or follow a motivational keto personality on Twitter or Instagram. Whatever you do, make sure that you have easy access to support during this journey. These actions become more critical if the people around you aren't onboard with keto. You may even consider planning a meetup with others who follow the keto lifestyle in your local area if you join a Facebook or other group. Check out our keto resources in Chapter 23 for good options.

TIP

Avoid apologizing for your change in eating habits. You're doing something great for your health, and apologizing for it subconsciously tells your friends — and yourself — that you're doing something wrong. This couldn't be further from the truth.

Talking with Your Doctor

Your doctor is the most knowledgeable person you know about nutrition and health, right? Not so fast. Not all medical doctors got adequate training in nutrition during medical school. Recently, a group of medical students at Bristol

University in the UK petitioned the college to include more nutrition information — it turns out, they get less than 25 hours of instruction across up to six years of medical training. Doctors just aren't trained in creating good health with food.

Although doctors know a lot about how insulin works in the body and the names of all the steps it takes to break down fat, they likely have less background on all of the research available regarding keto and its benefits. Many doctors may even equate keto with the Atkins diet, and could fall back on old dogmas: Grains are best and you need to limit your cholesterol to less than 300 milligrams a day. Luckily, more doctors are reading the new research on keto and opening up to the fact that there are tremendous benefits to a low-carb lifestyle.

TIP

If your doctor isn't up to date on research regarding keto, let him or her know frankly about your diet shift and why you're making the change. Offer to provide some research (doctors are scientists and love facts!) to help get him or her onboard. Let your improved health speak for itself. If you lose more weight than you have on a low-fat diet, if you're able to cure yourself of persistent acne, if you can reduce your dosage and perhaps even cut out some diabetes medications, remind your doctor that the major change you've made is keto and it's the reason for the improvement in your overall health.

Be aware that as you commit to the keto lifestyle, some of your routine blood tests may change; if you — and your doctor — don't realize that these are the result of your dietary changes, a lot of frustration may occur due to misinformation. Keto has just gone mainstream over the past couple of years, and many physicians may be unaware that blood tests will differ in people on keto compared to people on a high-carbohydrate diet. The difference in your blood tests may represent a new "normal" of keto even if it falls outside of the range that most doctors are familiar with.

For example, a "normal" heart rate is between 60 and 100 beats per minute. However, it's well-known that highly trained athletes, such as marathon runners, tend to have a slower heart rate — often in the 40s or 50s, and sometimes as low as the 30s. This would be pretty alarming if you just saw the number and didn't know the context. Obviously, an elite athlete's slow heart rate isn't a sign of disease; her heart is functioning normally based on her body's physiology. The truth is that her heart is so functionally capable that it can do the same amount of work in half the number of beats that it would take a more sedentary person's heart to accomplish.

In the same way, healthy changes from the keto lifestyle may show up as "abnormal" test results when they actually indicate that your body is improving its function. For example, when you're on keto, your doctor may notice that your LDL ("bad" cholesterol) is rising, but it will be accompanied by an increase in HDL ("good" cholesterol) and decrease in triglycerides (free-floating fat in your bloodstream), which is more important to your overall heart health than just focusing on the rise in LDL. The increase in LDL is probably a rise in the less-harmful intermediate and large, buoyant LDL, which doesn't have a substantial impact on your heart health anyway (see Chapter 4). If you educate yourself on these changes, you won't assume that the adjustments in your test results indicate that going keto was a mistake.

Another common "abnormal" finding on keto is a drop in active thyroid hormone level. You may have heard that keto can cause hypothyroidism. This is a bit of a complicated issue. It's well documented that people who lose weight — which often happens on keto — tend to have lower thyroid hormone levels. That's because the thyroid hormone increases your metabolism, the opposite of what the body wants when it's going through a period of weight loss. It's also why it can be challenging to continue to lose weight when you start — your thyroid activity drops, and your body holds on to any excess fat with a vicelike grip.

On the other hand, undergoing a stressful life situation can unmask an underlying thyroid problem. Sudden or extreme weight loss, illness, and even a drastic change to your eating habits, can put extra stress on your body. An extreme case of keto flu can definitely be a stressor. If you notice a prolonged keto flu that doesn't really get better over a week or so, or increasing fatigue, hair loss, or feeling cold all the time, this may be a thyroid problem. If you experience these symptoms, it's a good idea to be evaluated by your doctor to determine what's going on.

Many people transitioning to keto recover from keto flu quickly — or don't even experience it. If you're one of the people on keto who doesn't have any problems in your health, it may be that a blood test showing a low thyroid level is just a new "normal" for you. Thyroid hormones can drop on keto, even when you aren't losing weight or don't have any symptoms of a slowed metabolism. In this case, your body may not need as much thyroid hormone to produce the same result. You can think of this as being similar to someone who has insulin sensitivity, rather than insulin insensitivity. No one is too concerned if your insulin levels are on the low side — it just means your body responds to low levels of insulin and doesn't need to ramp up its production to have an effect. In the same way, if your thyroid hormones are low, but you have no symptoms of thyroid disease, it's unlikely you have a real problem — your body may merely be responding to thyroid hormones appropriately.

TIP

If your doctor is unfairly opposed to nutritional changes or is unwilling to accept your choice to go keto, consider looking for someone who is more open to talking about nutrition and its effect on health. This may be more important if you have a medical condition that requires care by a doctor. You can find resources for keto-friendly doctors at www.lowcarbusa.org/low-carb-providers/lchf-doctors.

4

Maximizing the Benefits

Consider fasting, find the best fasting method for you, and avoid fasting pitfalls.

Know how keto will impact your exercise routine and adapt your workouts to keto.

Chapter **12**

Fasting

Y ou've probably heard of intermittent fasting as a common practice for celebrities who need a drastic makeover before their next movie. Fasting is not only excellent for fat loss and muscle gains, but it also has a wide range of other health benefits.

Before we delve into the many benefits of fasting, we should talk about what fasting is and what it isn't. *Fasting* is voluntary abstinence from food (when it's available) for health, spiritual, or a host of other personal reasons. It is *not* starvation, because your food source is not unstable, and it is also not avoiding eating out of a fear of gaining excess body weight. Of course, fasting requires listening to your body and being aware of hunger cues — when it's time to break your fast because your body has reached a limit — and not pushing it to the point of starving your body (voluntarily or not) of the nutrients it needs.

Eating on a schedule is a modern, made-up luxury. Humans have a long history of prolonged periods of not eating. For millennia, our Paleolithic ancestors ate when they had the opportunity, not because it was lunchtime. Although this eating pattern wasn't exactly voluntary, they adapted to it, and it became the lifestyle. They likely ate more foods that were closer to a keto regimen — there were no Dunkin Donuts or breakfast cereals available, after all. They had occasional meat (with protein and fat) and a few plants and berries available that were probably higher in fiber than refined carbs. That led to hours or even days of no food consumption at all. They were able to survive these periods of "fasting" because their bodies were likely keto-adapted, used to burning fat for fuel both when there was and wasn't any food available, so there wasn't a significant shift in their metabolism during the periods of feast and famine. They were the original intermittent fasters, and they did it without a second thought.

Luckily, ketosis and fasting go hand in hand. If you're in ketosis, your body is already burning fat for fuel, which makes it that much easier to continue to do so when you go into fasting mode. If you're eating a standard American diet and you suddenly decide to fast, it'll be much harder because your body has to shift from burning carbs before it can get into fat burning. That means drops in blood sugar levels, mood swings, and feeling "hangry," which would make it less likely for you to be able to commit to fasting.

Recognizing the Benefits of Fasting

Scientists are discovering tons of benefits to intermittent fasting. Although the discoveries are new, we as a species have been doing it for millennia. Researchers are just finally catching up to what we've naturally been doing and identifying that it's a good idea to go back to ancient ways of eating.

Keto and intermittent fasting are the perfect marriage of healthy nutrition, and intermittent fasting may take your keto to the next level. In this section, we take a look at how intermittent fasting can help improve your keto lifestyle results.

Accelerating fat loss

Ketosis helps with fat loss by transforming your body into a fat-burning machine. Adding intermittent fasting to ketosis will accelerate fat loss. As we discuss in Chapter 3, no matter where you start off, if you stop eating for long enough, your body will stop burning glucose and instead switch to the more efficient fat and ketone burning associated with ketosis and long periods of abstinence from food. This is so important because of insulin, which regulates blood sugar levels. When you fast, you increase your sensitivity to insulin, those hormone levels drop, and you're less likely to do what high insulin tells your body to do: Burn glucose and store fat.

When carbs (and, therefore, insulin to a large degree) is out of the picture, as is the case with fasting, your body can burn fat, rather than store it. Most important, you can keep it off. The keto diet helps to decrease overall insulin levels, but even keto-approved food (the small number of carbs and the protein) will cause a slight increase in insulin levels after you eat. Fasting does away with that because food is what triggers insulin levels to rise. When you fast, your insulin levels drop, and this triggers your body to burn fat for a more extended period.

Many of these changes are likely maintained by a "fasting hormone," *adiponectin*. Adiponectin is increased with calorie restriction, fasting, and weight loss, even though — surprisingly — it's made by fat cells. Adiponectin has a host of beneficial effects that may explain some of the advantages of intermittent fasting. Higher adiponectin levels are associated with weight loss, whereas low levels are found in individuals who struggle with insulin resistance and type 2 diabetes. In fact, one of the medicines used to treat type 2 diabetes works to increase the levels of adiponectin in the body.

Here's some of what adiponectin does:

>> Decreases fat storage in your body and helps you lose weight

>> Stops the release of free fatty acids in the bloodstream and may help reduce inflammation

>> Stops glucose production from the liver and increases insulin sensitivity

>> Decreases your risk of diabetes and obesity

Studies have repeatedly demonstrated this: A review of overweight people who reduced calorie intake or fasted — without calorie counting — lost the same amount of weight.

Although both fasting and keto help reduce insulin levels, fasting accentuates keto. When you eat a keto diet, you're providing fat for your body to burn, and it will burn fat from food before it turns to stored body fat. When you burn through the food you've eaten, however, your digestive system begins to work off of stored fat. The longer your fasting period lasts, the more time you're giving yourself to work through stored fat. The human body can have tens of thousands of calories stored as fat, and if you want your body to use those calories, intermittent periods of fasting are a proven way to achieve your goal.

There are other hormones apart from adiponectin and insulin that are important for fat loss and are affected by what you do — or don't — put in your body:

>> **Ghrelin:** Ghrelin is often considered the "feeding hormone" (other common names are the growth, growing, or hunger hormone — it basically tells you to eat more!). It's made in the stomach and is a short-term mechanism for telling our body what and how much to eat. It's the hormone that increases right before you dig into lunch and minimizes your ability to burn calories. It also grows your fat cells (partially by increasing the release of growth hormone) and helps your stomach prepare for more food. Losing weight decreases ghrelin levels, and amounts in the blood may be related to the size of your stomach.

>> **Leptin:** This hormone work in the opposite way that ghrelin works and is considered the "satiety hormone." Like adiponectin, leptin is made from fat cells. It tells your body that you've had enough and increases your metabolism. Its levels rise with food intake, discouraging you from overdoing it at the bread buffet. In the long term, levels of leptin vary: Thin people have lower levels, while overweight people have higher levels. This may seem counterintuitive (more is better, right?), but similar to high levels of insulin that stop having the intended benefit, overweight individuals become desensitized to the hormone, getting "leptin insensitivity" so that they don't experience as much of an effect from leptin. This leads to more weight gain despite high levels of the hormone.

Studies show the interaction between these hormones plays a significant role in energy metabolism. Ghrelin tends to make it really challenging to lose weight, while leptin can increase your ability to drop pounds. In the same way, elevated adiponectin helps burn calories as it improves your insulin sensitivity. Fasting is a time-honored tradition that can positively affect all these hormones to help you feel your best.

Despite what many people think, fasting can actually help peak your metabolism. Prolonged starvation may do the opposite, but over the short term of a fast (several days), the body's level of adrenaline (or epinephrine) goes up. Adrenaline is part of the fight-or-flight system. You don't want adrenaline to be chronically elevated, but in the short term it can be highly beneficial. Short bursts of adrenaline lead to increased energy use, even when you're fasting. Adrenaline increases the release of any stored glucose you have available and enhances your ability to burn fat. Studies show that during a short, four-day fast, basal metabolism can increase by up to 12 percent, which can fuel weight loss.

Boosting muscle gain

Fasting can help improve muscle gains in a few ways. We walk you through them in this section.

Boosting human growth hormone

Human growth hormone (HGH) causes development and growth in children and teenagers. Of course, it's normal during this time in anyone's life to increase muscle mass naturally. Unfortunately, HGH tends to drop after you reach the end of your teenage years, and it never quite picks up again. HGH levels are almost twice as high in children and teenagers as they are in adults. HGH is a *pulsatile* hormone, meaning that its levels spike and decline. HGH has multiple effects:

>> Increases muscle mass

>> Increases bone strength and growth

>> Breaks down fat

>> Increases protein synthesis

>> Increases gluconeogenesis in the liver

>> Increases growth of all the organs (apart from the brain)

Studies show that providing shots of HGH to both men and women increased muscle mass and bone density while decreasing fat. HGH has been popular as a doping agent in elite sports, and some athletes have used it since the 1980s to improve their athletic abilities. Sadly, injecting HGH comes with a list of side effects like high blood sugar and risk for some cancers and heart issues. Luckily, fasting provides a natural burst of HGH without any of its nagging side effects. Eating suppresses HGH and overeating — or snacking — makes it plummet.

Cleaning house

Another way fasting improves muscle mass is by accentuating the cell's ability to regulate its daily cleaning cycle. Similar to your computer's virus system, your cells are continually monitoring their surroundings for any defects and will repair any abnormal processes. There are two systems that your cells use to do this:

>> **Autophagy lysosome:** This is literally "self-eating" and is the process of gobbling up long-lived (and often abnormal) proteins, RNA molecules, and cellular parts such as the mitochondria, which is the "powerhouse" of the cell. A specific type of autophagy, called *macroautophagy,* helps reduce metabolic and oxidative stress and is vital for the ability of proteins and other cell parts to be recycled for energy.

>> **Ubiquitin proteasome:** This is the principal mechanism for breaking down and recycling short-lived protein in all your cells. This system is vital for making sure your immune system is functioning, as well as repairing your DNA, the set of blueprints that encodes life. If this system is abnormal, it can lead to a host of diseases like neuromuscular degeneration and immune problems.

These pathways work together to repair your body's cells. Cells are complex, with multiple moving parts, like proteins and mitochondria that power each cell and serve as messengers to carry out essential functions. Whenever a part malfunctions, it must be repaired so the whole cell doesn't suffer. If either pathway is blocked, the cell becomes damaged, ultimately leading to cell death or destruction.

In muscle cells, this can lead to muscle weakness and wasting. Because muscles are highly active, lengthening and contracting many times a minute, they can easily get worn out if the tools to monitor or repair them are damaged. Besides, maintaining muscle requires a delicate balance of *muscle protein synthesis* (the scientific term for how muscles grow) and muscle breakdown. These pathways are stimulated by fasting and are a vital part of the body's ability to maintain muscle function.

Exciting new research shows that autophagy is necessary to maintain muscle mass, and without it, you're likely to lose the muscle you've worked hard to achieve slowly. Studies of animals stripped of the autophagy-promoting gene developed *muscular dystrophy* — a disease in which the muscles shrink over time, becoming progressively weaker, and eventually leading to difficulty walking, standing, and doing all the routine activities of daily life.

Your muscles won't necessarily disappear if you don't start fasting, but this research suggests that if you don't boost autophagy — effectively accomplished by fasting — you risk increasing muscle loss, setting you up for negative consequences, such as increased likelihood of disability and a loss of independence.

REMEMBER

Intermittent fasting has often been popularized by highly trained athletes, who prioritize a sculpted and lean physique. It would be surprising if they continued to fast if they lost muscle mass or saw a decrease in their performance. Their results indicate that fasting works for a lot of people.

Accelerating recovery and repair

Fasting helps to keep the body in good working order. Fasting can improve your body's function by

>> Decreasing oxidative damage to the body's proteins

>> Decreasing oxidative damage to DNA

>> Decreasing the accumulation of dysfunctional proteins and parts of cells

Fasting not only affects insulin and glucose levels, but also exerts a significant effect on a closely related hormone, *insulin-like growth factor 1* (IGF-1). IGF-1 is stimulated by HGH and causes most of the adverse effects of excess HGH, like high blood sugar and the risk of cancers. IGF-1 is mostly made by the liver and helps promote the growth of almost all the cells in both children and adults, from muscles to bones.

Excess IGF-1 is tightly linked to an increased risk of cancers, a condition characterized by the inability of the body to regulate and repair abnormal cells. There are multiple checkpoints throughout a cell's life that allow for evaluation, repair, and even the death of cells that have lost function — or worse, are becoming abnormal or cancerous. IGF-1 decreases the body's ability to manage these abnormal cells. Interestingly enough, people with IGF-1 deficiency are extremely unlikely to get cancer. Research shows that the blood from people with IGF-1 deficiency may protect cells from undergoing oxidative DNA damage. And even if some cells became damaged, the IGF-1 blood helped to make sure the cells were destroyed or discarded so they wouldn't grow to form cancer.

More research is needed, but small studies show that people who fast while taking advanced medication for cancer, such as chemotherapy, may do better than people who merely receive the chemotherapy. Not only do the people on fasts notice fewer side effects from chemotherapy — of which there are many — but studies show that in mice, intermittent fasting can decrease the risk of blood cancers and may be just as effective as chemotherapy for certain types of cancers.

Interestingly, fasting-induced autophagy is inhibited by *mammalian target of rapamycin* (mTOR), one of the common complexes that are upregulated during cancer and one of the primary targets for cancer drugs. This is more proof that natural ways to boost autophagy may help reduce our risk of cancer, or even treating it after it has formed. In addition to decreasing the risk of neurodegenerative disorders like Alzheimer's, fasting-induced autophagy helps limit inflammation throughout the body, which is also useful for reducing susceptibility to cancer (because many cancers are thought to be related to increased inflammation).

Improving skin tone

Clear skin may not be the first benefit you think of when fasting is mentioned, but it can be a particularly enticing bonus. Similar to keto's effect on acne, intermittent fasting may produce better results than a ten-part skincare regimen or a few extra hours of beauty rest. The key to fasting's benefit to your skin is the significant amount of anti-inflammation that is happening throughout your body. Your skin is the largest organ you have, and when your body is healthy, your skin will naturally follow suit.

Inflammation and stress naturally show up early on the skin, and fasting — in a healthy manner, with an adequate amount of water — is a great way to relieve stress throughout the body. While autophagy is working its magic to improve muscle health and to maintain nutrition in the brain, fasting allows the digestive system to rest and increases the billions of healthy bacteria in the gut. A well-functioning gut is vital for beautiful skin, because the digestive system has the highest number of immune cells of any part of the body. Optimal immunity will make sure that your skin is able to stop blackheads and acne in their tracks and help reduce the fine lines and wrinkles associated with aging.

This finding is not just anecdotal to people who fast for religious or health reasons. Research reveals the benefit of fasting on a host of skin ailments:

>> **Studies show that intermittent fasting helps improve wound healing in mice and also improves the thickness of their fur and improves blood supply to the skin.** Fasting also helps to decrease damage to the proteins in the skin that happen as we age, lower abnormal metabolites that build up in the skin over time and lead to wrinkles, tighten sagging skin, and even minimize age spots.

>> **Fasting may work synergistically with any skincare regimen you have.** Another study showed that fasting while using a topical *retinoid* (a common ingredient in skincare products that causes a lot of irritation to many users) decreased the rate of side effects while maintaining the benefits of retinol on the skin.

>> **Fasting may also lower the risk of inflammatory skin conditions like eczema and psoriasis.** In a study where individuals completed an intermittent fasting regimen, researchers observed a decrease in skin inflammation over a period of just two weeks, while another study showed regression of psoriatic plaques. Still another study showed the resolution of active whiteheads in people who have acne by improving skin oiliness and opening pores. Fasting reduces *sebum* (the oil that clogs the skin pores) by up to 40 percent, and with it, acne!

REMEMBER

Another critical part of a fast is drinking plenty of water. It's important to remember that we're encouraging water fasting, instead of a dry fast in which nothing — including water — is consumed. When all you have to take in is water — and the occasional non-caloric fluids — you tend to maintain your fluid levels. Drinking water and staying hydrated is crucial for skin health, and water fasts encourage this.

Slowing the aging process

Fasting can help you live longer. As fasting improves the body's ability to heal and recover from negative events like disease and infection, the body is much more likely to thrive over the long term. This increased health is related to the body's ability to oppose disease. Insulin and glucose, which drop when you fast, are strongly associated with disease and rapid aging. Fasting for about three days decreases blood levels of both by about 30 percent. IGF-1, the downstream effector of HGH, can also accelerate aging. Yet, fasting drops IGF-1 by up to 60 percent. Interestingly, this benefit is partially due to protein restriction, suggesting that fasting works in different ways from keto to improve long-term health.

Fasting reduces inflammation and improves the cells' ability to heal. Fasting works its magic by promoting autophagy and a host of other hormone actors that help to decrease infection, illness, and disease, all of which are associated with aging at a cellular level.

Many scientists believe that the telomere is essentially the epitome of the body's fountain of youth. *Telomeres* are the protective cap at the end of chromosomes that protect chromosomes from unraveling. Because chromosomes are the blueprint of bodies and brains, short telomeres are more likely to lead to disease and aging because damaged chromosomes aren't able to write out foolproof instructions to maintain a healthy body and mind. The length of telomeres decreases as you age — and it's one reason scientists believe that people have a higher risk for disease, infections, and even cancer as they age.

Because fasting increase the cells' ability to promote autophagy, and autophagy is a known factor in elongating telomeres, fasting is conclusively linked to a reduction in aging. Also, autophagy and telomeres are related in another way. The enzyme that increases telomere length — telomerase — also boosts cellular autophagy. In this way, autophagy and telomeres have a symbiotic relationship.

REMEMBER

Studies show that long-term fasting — generally more than 24 hours — is needed to get the benefits of autophagy, and that's why some authorities suggest a benefit of occasional long-term fasts of three or more days. Most people have to work their way up slowly to this goal, and some people should only do this under the supervision of a healthcare professional. If you have any preexisting medical condition, make sure to speak with your doctor before beginning any fasting routine.

Improving brain function

A commonly voiced concern is that fasting will lower the ability to think and accomplish necessary day-to-day obligations, but the opposite often happens. There are countless reports of people noticing that they feel sharper and more alert the longer they go into a fast. The first time you fast may be difficult because your body isn't used to being without calories, but as it adjusts you may notice mental clarity that you've missed for a long time.

This makes sense: If humans had evolved to get brain fog whenever they were hungry, they never would've survived as a species. Can you imagine if our ancestors got more and more lethargic on the second or third day without food that they would have survived to the fourth day when they needed all their wits about them to catch dinner? Instead, their reaction times stayed sharp, their vision was excellent, and their mental clarity was never better. It's more likely that they were most vulnerable those first few hours after having a satisfying dinner — likely similar to the post-Thanksgiving energy crash that you're probably familiar with.

With a full stomach, energy is diverted toward digestion of a large number of calories, and humans are neither as alert nor focused as when they're hungry.

Interestingly, humans — and other mammals — have evolved so that low-calorie intake or fasting does not affect brain size. Most people, if they fast long enough (we're talking about weeks without eating), will begin to notice muscle, bone, and other organs deteriorate. However, brain size will stay stable longer than anything else. This is crucial because your brain is your most potent asset. Outsmarting a predator was the best way to survive — because our ancestors were definitely not the largest or strongest animals in the jungle. Therefore, they were much more likely to survive than if their brain cells didn't start to peter out as soon as they got hungry.

This is where the benefit of a keto/intermittent-fasting combination comes in. The brain needs some glucose to survive, even if you're not consuming any carbohydrates. The liver can use gluconeogenesis to convert protein to glucose, meeting the brain's needs even in an environment devoid of carbs. Studies show that with absolutely no food, your body and brain could survive for about 30 days. The rest of you will definitely shrink, but your body will prioritize nutrients going to your brain to keep your mind as sharp as possible until you eat again.

Fasting — and exercise — also have direct benefits on the growth and function of brain cells and neurons. Studies show that both calorie restriction and fasting increase the activity of neurons in the hippocampus, a vital brain center for learning and memory. These neurons release brain-derived neurotrophic factor (BDNF), which improves the brain's function through several mechanisms:

>> Growing and maintaining the *dendrites* of neurons, which are the finger-like extensions of neurons that allow them to receive input from other parts of the brain.

>> Developing and maintaining *synapses,* the spaces between neurons that are vital for communication between different neurons in the same and different parts of the brain.

>> Allowing for the development and growth of neurons from brain *stem cells,* the ancestors of neurons that have the potential to become any type of cell within the brain. This allows for the growth of even more neurons to improve connections and increase brain function.

Alzheimer's disease often attacks the neurons of the hippocampus, leading to dementia and forgetfulness, but fasting may be a way to prevent the progressive decline of Alzheimer's by fortifying the brain cells most susceptible to disease. In fact, both BDNF and insulin seem to be inversely related to drops in cognitive ability. Studies show that rats that were fed twice a day and were otherwise on an intermittent fasting routine did better running through mazes and other tasks that require a working memory than rats that could eat whenever they wanted.

Reducing inflammation

Most of the diseases in the modern age are related to inflammation. Whether cancer, heart disease, autoimmune disease, pain syndromes, or a host of other conditions, they all can be traced back to underlying inflammation in the body. This has led many nutritionists and doctors to search high and low for an "anti-inflammatory diet" that would help cure society of the ills that are affecting health and life span. Research shows that the best anti-inflammatory diet may well be fasting.

Individuals who fast long term (between one and three weeks at a time) have experienced benefits that are atypical for many conventional medical treatments and procedures. Here are two such examples:

>> **Rheumatoid arthritis (RA):** RA is an autoimmune form of arthritis that can be even more devastating than osteoarthritis. In both animal and human models of the disease, fasting can cause remission that lasts two years or longer. This is in the face of a usually chronically progressive disease that leaves sufferers unable to use their hands merely to button their shirts or open jars.

>> **Hypertension (high blood pressure):** This is commonly known as the "silent killer," but its condition can improve by following a keto diet. This change often requires a consistent and long-term commitment, however. On the other hand, in only 13 days of water-only fast, individuals with borderline high blood pressure dropped blood pressure readings by 20 points. Even more exciting, in people with a diagnosis of high blood pressure, a prolonged fast of 10 or 11 days led to completely normal blood pressures that dropped between 40 and 60 points. This result is better than what is typically seen in years of treatment with blood pressure medicines.

Of course, type 2 diabetes is, at its core, an inflammatory condition and associated with the metabolic syndrome, a combination of five diseases that are all based on inflammation:

>> Obesity (mainly when it's around your waist)

>> High blood pressure

>> Insulin insensitivity (or high blood sugar)

>> High triglycerides (the free fatty acids roaming around your bloodstream)

>> Cholesterol problems (unusually low levels of high-density lipoprotein [HDL], the good kind of cholesterol)

Fasting can help address all these issues. Alternate-day fasting seems to be an excellent approach when dealing with any of these conditions. When people either drastically cut their calories every other day (to between nothing and as much as 500 to 600 calories per day), blood pressure drops, waistlines shrink, and they regain sensitivity to insulin. Various studies showed this effect in both overweight and healthy-weight people and took as little as a 15-day to a three-week commitment to alternate-day fasting. Daily intermittent fasting works as well. A study looking at practicing Muslims with metabolic syndrome who fasted from sunrise to sunset for the month of Ramadan found lower glucose levels, as well as improved insulin sensitivity over time.

An underlying mechanism for this is autophagy and fasting's effect on *Sirtuin 1* (SIRT1), an enzyme that helps to block inflammation throughout your body. SIRT1 turns off many genes that are important for increasing stress-related inflammation, which may be one of the early triggers of cancer. Also, it helps to stabilize proteins and make them able to function longer, so your body doesn't have to waste energy on new protein production. By working together, SIRT1 and autophagy help maintain cell integrity while reducing waste.

Another mechanism is *adiponectin,* the "starvation hormone," which is boosted by fasting. Adiponectin is likely also anti-inflammatory because it helps to reverse the early stages of *atherosclerotic* heart disease (the kind where the arteries are clogged). Higher adiponectin levels decrease the inflammatory molecules that make up plaque, which causes arteries to harden and can ultimately lead to a heart attack. Studies have also shown that adiponectin may protect the liver from damage.

Detoxing cells

To heal and be effective, the body has to go through natural periods of detoxification. This is more efficient and healthier than any detox diet you can do and is entirely self-sufficient. However, the effectiveness of this natural process can decrease as you age. Intermittent fasting to the rescue!

Christian de Duve, the 1974 Nobel Prize winner, realized how cells detox through a process called *autophagy.* Cells have *lysosomes,* essentially garbage disposal units that periodically search the cell for any damaged or abnormal parts that need to be fixed or removed so that the whole cell doesn't become cancerous or damaged. This process is autophagy (literally meaning "self-eating"), and it's the cell's way of continually renewing itself. Autophagy is an integral part of the body's work, but it's inhibited by

- » Insulin
- » Glucose
- » Protein

The common factor of these three things is eating. Even if you're following a keto diet, moderate protein will stop autophagy, and the small number of low-carb foods will affect it. There is no possible way of eating that will induce autophagy; however, some diets, like keto, may encourage its natural process more than others. When insulin levels rise, or amino acids from the digested pieces of your steak arrive in your bloodstream, this signals your body that more nutrients are coming in and old worn-out cells don't need to be refurbished to produce energy. That means eating anything — even a ketogenic diet — regularly will block autophagy. Only fasting can combat this.

Yoshinori Ohusmi, a 2016 Nobel Prize winner, furthered the understanding of how the process works, revealing that autophagy is vital in

- » Preventing cancer
- » Cell survival
- » Quality control of organs of every part of the cell
- » Body-wide metabolism
- » Management of inflammation and immunity

These are essential parts of how the body works and thrives, and fasting is able to turn up all these mechanisms so that they work at their optimal level. Another benefit of autophagy is that it keeps the brain in its best shape. Alzheimer's disease, one of the most common neurodegenerative brain disorders in humans, happens when the brain is filled with an abnormal protein, called *amyloid beta*. This abnormal protein destroys the connections between brain cells, leading to difficulty with memory and learning. Autophagy tends to remove this abnormal protein, decreasing its ability to accumulate and lead to Alzheimer's disease. Studies also show that fasting can help minimize the traumatic effects of

- » Epileptic seizures
- » Stroke
- » Traumatic brain injury
- » Spinal cord injuries

REMEMBER

There are so many benefits to intermittent fasting that the better question to ask may be, "Are there any benefits to snacking?"

Sampling Different Fasting Methods

Fasting is not a one-size-fits-all method. Just like each keto follower is different in terms of go-to proteins or favorite fats, your intermittent fasting may be different from another healthy person's. There is no specific definition of fasting, although studies suggest that a minimum of 16 hours between meals is needed to get the benefits of reduced inflammation and an increase in autophagy (see "Detoxing cells," earlier in this chapter for more on autophagy).

There are several options for fasting. You can opt for a "time-restricted" schedule or alternate-day fasting. In the time-restricted option, you eat only during a set number of hours of the day, whether it's four hours or eight. On the other hand, during alternate-day fasting, you'll stop eating for a full 24 hours, so you eat one day and fast the next, or you choose certain days during the week to fast. Some people also choose a "modified" fast in which, rather than fasting, they decrease their calories drastically on the "fasted" day, generally to about 20 percent to 25 percent of their regular caloric intake.

Read on to look at the most common options for intermittent fasting — and remember that some people choose to switch between different styles or incorporate multiple types of fasting into their nutrition routine.

The 16-hour fast

The most popular time-restricted feeding method was developed by the well-known Swedish bodybuilder and personal trainer Martin Berkhan, who dubbed it the "Leangains" method. His method allows you to eat for 8 hours during the day and fast for the remaining 16 hours. This intermittent fasting is highly tied to workouts, and Berkhan touts it as a way to gain muscle while losing fat. As such, simply doing intermittent fasting without the exercise part will be unlikely to provide all the "leangains" that he suggests.

Because you can choose to be sleeping for a significant part of the "fasted time," this option is very doable option for many people. You can technically choose any 16-hour period to be your fasted time, but most people fast through the night and start eating around noon. However, if you go to bed or wake up significantly earlier or later than most, it's fine to shift your "feeding period" as best you see fit. Generally, with this setup, your first meal should be the largest — and come after a workout. The size and caloric content of your meals gradually decreases over the following eight hours, although if you choose to work out late in the day, you may eat your most substantial meal after that workout.

TIP

A crucial cornerstone of this method is that your most substantial meal happens after you work out. Martin also recommends keeping to your schedule, whatever it is. We're creatures of habit, so if you plan on sticking to this schedule, it'll be easier to maintain it if your feeding period is always around noon to 8 p.m. instead of shifting it to morning/afternoon or evening/night depending on your plans for the day.

Generally, Martin encourages a high-protein diet at all times, with higher fats when you aren't working out and higher carbs when you are. The Leangains method is actually based on quite a bit of evidence from studies that looked at its effect on both humans and mice, showing that 16 hours is the minimum amount of time needed to initiate the benefits of fasting. Also, studies show that most people can adhere to this diet because there is a substantial enough period in which you can eat through your waking hours.

One meal a day

The 20-hour fast, or "warrior diet," was developed by a man named Ori Hofmekler in 2001. He coined the term based on the ancient Spartan warriors who historians believe ate little during the day — and worked out plenty — and then feasted at night after the battle was over. Ori believed that the long fast would stress the body into becoming lean and healthy, similar to what happened to our ancient ancestors.

Compared to the Leangains method (see the preceding section), the warrior diet has much less scientific backing. Still, because it does use a time-restricted method of fasting, which has proven benefits in shorter stretches, it isn't unreasonable to think that a 20-hour fast would also provide benefits.

One small study that lasted six months did look at 20-hour fasting periods during the day and found that participants experienced both fat loss and muscle gains. Not surprisingly, the people who ate for only four hours felt subjectively much hungrier than the control group. Surprisingly, they also had higher blood pressure readings, although their cortisol levels were reduced.

Hofmekler's method does allow you to eat a small number of low-calorie foods like raw veggies and hard-boiled eggs during the 20-hour "fast" to get you through the day, and then you can gorge during the four hours of eating. You're encouraged to feast on whole, unprocessed foods, but there are no real restrictions on what you can and can't eat during the feasting hours.

Interestingly, some studies do show that the time you eat does make a difference. Although the warrior diet typically has you eating your largest meal in the evening, some studies show there is a benefit to eating similar to the Mediterranean culture where the majority of calories are taken in during lunch, and there is a significant drop in calories toward the end of the day.

Research supports this approach via several mechanisms:

>> Insulin levels may be higher at night, meaning that you'll be more likely to store fat if you eat late.

>> HGH is suppressed overnight when you eat late, which is a potent stimulus for muscle growth (and improved metabolism).

>> Eating late can decrease your ability to get a good night's sleep as energy is diverted toward digesting your food.

>> Because ghrelin is naturally lower at night, you're actually overriding a natural tendency to eat less by eating late.

5-2 regimen

This kind of fast was popularized by Michael Mosely as the "Fast Diet." On this diet, participants eat normally five days a week and then commit to a 24-hour fast twice during the week. You're allowed to eat between 500 and 600 calories on the "fasting day," so it isn't technically a true "fast," but because it's a significant caloric restriction, it's considered to be beneficial. And some people choose to make the two days a true fast. Either way, the goal is to make this a long-term way of eating rather than a short-term plan for weight loss.

As opposed to "time-restricted feeding," fasting longer than 24 hours is considered *prolonged fasting*. This comes from research showing that, in mice, simply skipping all calories for at least a day was just as effective as significant calorie restriction in a number of areas; these included encouraging weight loss, improving insulin and glucose levels, and lowering overall cholesterol levels. There is less research on prolonged fasting in humans because it can be a bit difficult to find people who are willing to commit to 24-hour and longer fasts voluntarily.

However, anecdotally, people who fast for this long note that hunger tends to decrease and the freedom from food can be quite liberating. Still, there is an increased risk of possible side effects, including hypoglycemia and low blood pressure, and it may be difficult for many people to comply with this type of diet long term. Besides, anyone with significant health concerns or who takes daily medication should touch base with his doctor before committing to any kind of prolonged fasting.

Alternate-day fasting

This is a more intense fasting regimen, where you fast every other day. Similar to the 5-2 regimen, some people have a meager number of calories on their fasting days. Some may choose to do this indefinitely, but this regimen tends to be a short-term diet for faster weight loss that you stop after reaching your goal weight. This method of fasting was popularized by Brad Pilon, in his book *Eat, Stop, Eat.*

Research has demonstrated that benefits of alternate-day fasting include an improvement in cardiovascular risk factors, as well as improvement in body composition. In a study of overweight individuals, alternate-day fasting over ten weeks allowed participants to decrease fat mass, as well as increase adiponectin. They also had lower levels of low-density lipoprotein (LDL) and triglycerides.

Reducing the Downside of Fasting with the Keto Diet

If you're interested in intermittent fasting, but you're worried about experiencing intense hunger, this section is for you. Here, we list a few common fasting pitfalls and tell you how to combat or even avoid the side effects.

Getting your mind right

Hunger really starts in the mind. It's no wonder that there is so much money in advertising to make people interested in eating. If you focus on people's brains, you'll be much more effective at changing eating habits than if you focused exclusively on their stomachs.

TIP

Like anything else, controlling your eating "clock" is a habit. If you start small and work at it, fasting will get easier. Begin with small intermittent fasting periods, and work your way up. Commit to stop eating at a particular time and choose an herbal tea or other noncaloric drink to get you through the evening. Fasting is extremely easy when you sleep, so it may be helpful to try to get to bed at a reasonable time when you commit to intermittent fasting.

Starting slow and building your fasting muscle

Of course, no one starts a foray into fasting with a weeklong fast; instead, take your time working toward a regular time-restricted feeding period, and slowly build up your stamina to 24-hour or longer fasts. As you take your time and fasting becomes a routine part of your life, you'll decide if you want to try longer fasts to see if they'll help you reach your health goals.

TIP

Increase your fasting period slowly — a 16-hour fast is a lot more manageable than a 20-hour fast.

Staying active

Make sure to keep busy and productive. Because hunger is mostly in your mind, keeping your mind focused on other things is crucial, whether you're working, exercising, or taking time to pursue the activities you enjoy. You'll probably find that, like us, you're at your most creative and productive during your fast, so don't waste this time daydreaming about lunch.

We often eat when we're bored, angry, irritated, or other times that are not really related to our need to be nourished. This is an optimal time to delve into whatever emotional issue is causing stress and try to resolve the core issue rather than break your fast.

Maintaining healthy keto changes

Don't make the mistake of assuming that all calorie limits are off during your eating window on a time-restricted fast. Spartans were able to feast during the night, but they burned a lot of calories fighting during the day. Unless you're in basic training or setting up camp at the gym, you'll need to have some control during your feeding times, and you must remember that you'll still need to stay on the standard keto diet and limit carbs when you do eat.

TIP

Be keto-adapted first. Keto makes it a lot easier to stick to fasting because both are based on increasing ketones. Fasting can be quite challenging on the standard American diet, because you'll notice a change in blood sugar and energy levels. If you're already keto-adapted, your body is ready to reap all the benefits of fasting because you're already used to burning ketones for fuel. You'll also avoid any massive changes in insulin levels, making controlling your eating more manageable.

Staying hydrated

It's okay to drink noncaloric fluids like coffee, tea, water, or broth, and chew sugar–free gum. This can help quite a bit if you feel the need to replace eating with something you can do with your mouth. Over time, you may feel less of a need to do this, but of course, you'll need to keep your fluid intake up to stay hydrated. Remember to limit diet sodas — they're filled with artificial sweeteners, which can actually increase your cravings for sugary food.

TIP

As you get more accustomed to fasting, thoughts of your next meal will take a backseat as leptin drops, and you're fully in control of your nutrient intake. (See "Accelerating fat loss," earlier in this chapter, for more on leptin.)

A RARE CAUTION: REFEEDING SYNDROME

Refeeding syndrome is a rare occurrence and can occur in people who fast for more than five days or in situations where prolonged malnutrition has occurred. As such it's not of much concern to the vast majority of people who fast for less than that. If you stop eating for more than five days, the level of the mineral phosphorous in your blood can become depleted. As you begin to eat again, insulin rises, which requires a baseline level of phosphorous.

Excess phosphorous resides in your bones and muscles, and your body will start to break down these two parts of your body to get at the phosphorous. Unfortunately, this can lead to heart arrhythmias, as well as significant shifts in body fluid. Low levels of potassium and magnesium can also worsen this condition, leading to cramps, tremors, confusion, and exacerbated heart arrhythmias.

To avoid this situation on a longer fast, make sure to add a daily multivitamin to your routine or drink bone broth or other liquids with added electrolytes. Keep up with some physical activities — even if it's just walking — to maintain strength in your bones and muscles.

Remember: Similar to the keto diet, intermittent fasting should be used under the guidance of a physician — or not at all — in pregnant or breastfeeding women, children, or anyone who is taking blood-sugar-lower medications or has preexisting medical conditions. Also, although fasting doesn't cause eating disorders, most individuals who are currently dealing — or have dealt — with an eating disorder should probably avoid intermittent or prolonged fasting.

Chapter **13**

Maintaining a Fitness Routine

Now that we've covered the key players in successfully adapting to keto — what to eat, when, and how much — it's vital to delve into what you'll be doing for the vast amount of time during the day when you *aren't* eating. That's right: Movement is vital to achieving your health goals, whether it's bulking up, slimming down, or just reducing your risk of diabetes. Exercise not only is helpful for losing weight and chiseling out a six-pack, but also improves your cardiovascular health, releases feel-good endorphins, and improves your sleep. It's no wonder that health authorities recommend people engage in physical activity every day, and it's always part of doctors' prescription for good health.

Yet there can be a lot of misinformation regarding the best way to use exercise to reach your goals. Should you focus on resistance training alone to gain muscle or focus exclusively on cardio for weight loss? What's the best mix of exercises, and how does your exercise regimen interact with keto? Should you work out on an empty stomach or eat a small meal? And what's the best way to build endurance? The questions are seemingly endless, and it can be difficult to know how to incorporate a change in your eating — keto — into this multifaceted regimen.

REMEMBER

When you eat a healthy, whole-foods keto diet, there is little risk that you'll lose muscle, power, or endurance, and the same goes if you're skillfully incorporating intermittent fasting into your regimen. The critical question, then, is what your goals are. Do you want to sculpt lean muscle, lose extra fat, or maintain what you already have?

Here, we delve into all of this and more, taking your unique goals and background into account to determine the best way to make keto and exercise work together to get you your best results. We've even included a couple workout regimens to help you on your way to building endurance or losing excess fat.

As any physical trainer will say when you show up for your workout, "Let's get this started!"

Anticipating the Impact of the Keto Diet on Exercise

Exercising and keto go hand in hand. We all know that the numerous benefits of a regular physical routine will only accentuate the benefits that keto has for health disease prevention and fat loss. In this section, we explain how to incorporate exercise during different parts of your keto journey.

Exercising while transitioning into keto

While you're transitioning into a keto lifestyle, some of the symptoms can be quite intense. However, when you get through that initial transition — with a little know-how — you'll love the benefits of keto on the other side.

Almost no one would recommend high- or even moderate-intensity workouts while you're going through the keto flu or any other period of feeling unwell during your keto transition, but people have a wide range of reactions to the keto transition, and the length of time these reactions last varies as well. Some people choose to cut carbs quickly, and working out and even fasting may be part of their plan to get to their goals. Others view getting to keto as a long-term destination and transition for weeks or months.

Regardless of which path you choose, even though you may notice ketones in your blood or urine tests in the first few weeks after transitioning, you may not be fully keto-adapted and may notice a drop in your performance and energy levels that are not necessarily permanent. This experience can be discouraging, but it's important to remember that your body is still transitioning, and it may take weeks for you to return to your regular level of exercise performance.

USING EXERCISE TO GET INTO KETOSIS FASTER

Some people transition into ketosis easily and even use exercise to help them get into ketosis more quickly. Because exercise helps burn up extra *glycogen* (compounded glucose molecules) in your muscle, this method is proven to push you into ketosis. In fact, we used this method ourselves, when we walked for several hours every day to burn up extra muscle glycogen during our transition.

If you want to use exercise during your transition to ketosis, make sure to do so at a low to moderate intensity, stay well hydrated, and keep up with your electrolytes (see Chapter 7).

However, there are certain downsides to exercising during the transition period, especially if you do so too strenuously:

- **Intense symptoms:** Keto flu is one of the most dreaded parts of transitioning to keto, and exercising during the transition to ketosis is a surefire way to increase your chance of getting keto flu. If at any point you notice telltale signs of weakness, muscle aches, or nausea, stop exercising and give yourself a break.

- **Dehydration:** If you're exercising hard during your transition, you put yourself at risk for dehydration. Remember that as the glucose and glycogen in your system are expended, you naturally lose water weight. Adding sweat to the equation may push you into dehydration, especially if you aren't adequately replenishing with fluids and electrolytes.

- **Doing too much:** If you go too hard in the gym while transitioning, you may assume that keto is not for you. Exercising makes the transition harder, and you'll likely notice a decrease in performance and endurance. Also, it can take weeks for your muscles to become efficient at burning fat over glucose, which can be discouraging if you're not expecting it. Just remember that this is a temporary experience and your body will thank you after you've fully transitioned.

If you experience keto flu or just have a lot of unpleasant symptoms during your transition, you may want to take a short break from exercise, or at least decrease the intensity of your workouts. This setback is only temporary, as your body transitions to fat burning and has to recalibrate fuel sources for your muscles.

Exercising when you've adapted to keto

Keto adaptation happens when your body is fully accustomed to using ketones as its primary source of fuel. This process can take several months or more and requires a steady state of ketones in your blood. Because there is a widespread notion that exercise must include carbs for high-level performance, some people may be concerned that dropping carbs could lead to a reduction in endurance or power.

The concern probably comes from the idea that muscles preferentially use carbohydrates — glucose — to contract to their best ability. Research dating back to the 1960s has found that muscles tire earlier if they don't have enough glycogen (the form of glucose that is stored in muscle tissue), and an athlete will tire quickly, leading to worse workouts and worse performance. Since then, exercise physiologists, sports trainers, and the average Joe have popularized the benefit of "carbing up" before, during, and even after exercise to make sure that the muscles' stores of glycogen were topped off and to improve the ability to recover post-workout.

However, this is only true if your muscles are not adapted to using an alternate source for fuel. An athlete who typically consumes carb-heavy pasta or sugary sports beverages before a workout routine will definitely notice a drop in performance if he chooses to forgo the carbs before his next lifting session at the gym or long-distance bike ride. In these carb-adapted athletes, high glycogen stores are necessary because their muscles aren't used to turning to the highly effective ketones for long-lasting energy. So, when they ask their muscles to perform high-intensity activities, they'll use more carbohydrates to fuel their muscles while minimizing their relative use of fat. Many exercise physiologists erroneously claim that high-level performance relies almost exclusively on carbohydrates because the athletes who were evaluated tended to be carb-heavy athletes.

The situation is entirely different in the average keto dieter whose body is a pro at using ketones to power muscles. The main ketone, beta-hydroxybutyrate (BHB), is the perfect alternative to glucose to fuel your brain and your muscles. In the keto-adapted individual, carbohydrates are a secondary source of fuel, and even as muscle activity increases, these individuals are able to use more fat to fuel their muscles. What you eat changes how your body behaves on a daily basis, including how it reacts to a workout.

In fact, some research suggests that continually carb loading — even if it's just around the time of exercise — may decrease your ability to use fat optimally during training.

In the 1980s, a classic study was performed that looked at five well-trained cyclists to evaluate keto-adapted performance in athletes. The results gave credence to the idea that keto adaptation can maintain performance status in highly trained athletes. In the study, the athletes ate a strict keto diet (less than 20 grams of carbohydrates per day) for four weeks and then served as their own controls — their performance on the keto diet was compared to their previous performance on a standard high-carbohydrate diet. Researchers showed that, at a little over 60 percent of their maximal activity, these highly trained athletes were able to ride longer (151 minutes versus 147 minutes) on the keto diet. Additionally, they relied less on glucose as a muscle fuel, had normal blood glucose levels, and were able to transition their muscle use to high and efficient levels of fat metabolism.

TECHNICAL STUFF

MEASURING THE INTENSITY OF A WORKOUT

Here are two critical terms regarding the intensity of a workout and how that affects your fuel sources:

- **Metabolic equivalent (MET):** The amount of oxygen you use in a minute when you're lying around on the sofa. It's essentially a marker of your metabolism, so your MET is different from your mom's MET or your buddy's MET. A person's MET depends on muscle mass, ambient temperature, food intake, and a host of other factors, but primarily weight and gender. This system isn't entirely accurate, and it's why you shouldn't completely trust those MET numbers you see on the treadmill — they're an estimate. However, many studies use this concept, so it's a good one to know. The Compendium of Physical Activities is an online resource (https://sites.google.com/site/compendiumofphysicalactivities) that identifies the MET for a number of exercises. For example, both general jazz dancing and weight training are considered to have an MET of 5 (or five times your baseline activity).

- **Maximal aerobic activity or maximal oxygen consumption:** The maximum MET that you can maintain (for a set amount of time) without losing strength or speed. If you can just barely eke out ten reps of a 150-pound deadlift, for example, that's your maximal aerobic activity. It's a great idea to figure out what your levels are so you can see what gains you're making over time. It's often the ultimate goal in most studies and is the product of how much blood your heart can pump out multiplied by the amount of oxygen your body uses over a set amount of time. Maximal aerobic power tends to be higher in men than women (by 10 percent to 20 percent) due to men's larger muscle volume, oxygen-carrying capacity, and contraction of the heart muscle. It also decreases as you age by about 10 percent each decade if you don't exercise.

REMEMBER

Although this is excellent information and shows that keto did not negatively affect highly trained athletes' performance, this study looked at only one type of exercise, and it was a sport that emphasizes endurance, where keto excels. Studies now have expanded to look at different types of physical activity based on the intensity and length of the workout. There are several forms of exercise you can participate in:

>> **Short sprints:** Short sprints are intense activities that can last less than 10 seconds. During this period, your muscle uses creatine phosphate, which is stored and easily available energy in your muscles. Most of the creatine phosphate in your body is in your muscles, where about 95 percent of your total body stores are found. Creatine phosphate is critical in making adenosine triphosphate (ATP), which is basically raw energy for your body. ATP is required to get your muscle to contract immediately without having to waste time breaking down other fuel sources like glucose, protein, or fat. Yet, it's only a short-term fix, and it generally only fuels muscles for about 10 seconds before reinforcements have to be called in. Under normal circumstances, the body does this preemptively before muscles fatigue and have to switch to other types of metabolism for fuel. Creatine phosphate is a big deal for short bursts of intense activity like weightlifting at maximal potential or sprinting a hundred meters. This is the energy source that most people use to produce muscle gains in terms of strength and muscle mass, as well as improved recovery.

>> **High-intensity training:** These are intense activities in which you go all out (between 60 percent and 80 percent of your maximum level) from 10 seconds to about 2 minutes. During this time, you use *anaerobic metabolism,* which is where your muscles burn fuel without using oxygen. While this is happening, your muscles build up lactic acid, a compound that leads to a sensation of burning and intense fatigue after you've pushed hard. If your muscles don't rest or can't switch out of anaerobic metabolism, lactic acid continues to build up and, not only do your muscles fatigue, but ultimately your muscles will lose strength and can even become damaged with overexposure.

One of the benefits of anaerobic metabolism is that it tends to burn more calories over the short term, translating to improvements in overall body metabolism. High-intensity interval training (HIIT), or on-and-off bursts of high-intensity exercise, allows you to continue this level of activity for longer periods of time, but only because of the short recovery period between each "interval" where your body is able to get rid of some of the lactic buildup during rest. HIIT-style workouts can include a range of activities such as weight lifting, running, swimming, or whatever you choose.

>> **Endurance activities:** Endurance activities are extended, steady-state activities greater than ten minutes that require less overall strength and are generally considered moderate in intensity. This may be up to 60 percent of

your total muscle strength (but it's typically between 35 percent and 50 percent, depending on your level of fitness). This classic style of exercise uses *aerobic metabolism.* Aerobic metabolism is much more efficient than anaerobic exercise because it produces a steady state of energy.

TECHNICAL STUFF

Aerobic metabolism occurs when carbs, fats, and proteins are broken down in the presence of oxygen. Essentially, this is how your body gets energy when you're breathing enough to sustain whatever you're doing for a long time (think of a marathon runner who can maintain the same pace for hours). When you can't get enough oxygen to maintain an activity for a long period (think sprinting), your body gets energy from anaerobic metabolism, which happens in the absence of oxygen. As you can imagine, you get exhausted very quickly and have to recover by breathing hard.

Whereas anaerobic metabolism produces only 2 ATP for every molecule of glucose burned, aerobic metabolism produces a whopping 38 ATP. Obviously, that's way more bang for your exercise buck. Yet, aerobic exercise can use all types of fuel, including fat. This is where keto adaption shines, because fat is a wonderful fuel for aerobic activity and produces all the energy needed to sustain these longer and less-intense workouts. Endurance activities range from walking to cycling and other typical cardio workouts.

Of course, your body is incredibly dynamic and can switch between these different types of exercise even in the same workout. So, for example, if you switch from a moderate intensity warm up to an interval sprint interspersed by a long jog, your muscles go from aerobic to anaerobic to sprints in one session.

Glucose (which you get from carbohydrates) is the best source of fuel for high-intensity endurance activities because even keto-adapted athletes will require glucose during these workouts, and the same is true for us average Joes. *Glycolysis* is the breakdown of readily available sugar to power your muscles while exercising strenuously. Still, even on a keto diet, the body is able to make glucose through the process of gluconeogenesis (see Chapter 2). That means that, on keto, your muscles still do have some glucose and glycogen stores to use for acute muscle needs. In fact, one study of elite runners and triathletes who only differed based on their diet (keto versus high-carb) had similar levels of maximal aerobic capacity, with the keto runners having a slightly higher level, even though this was not significant. Whether you're a weekend warrior or training hard five times a week, you'll likely experience similar results.

On the other hand, muscles are able to use other sources, such as ketones, for short sprints and endurance-type activities. This process is called *fat oxidation,* and it's a process that breaks down fat to produce muscle contractions.

In the same study, the keto-adapted athletes were able to use fat an average of 2.3 times better than the high-carb runners to fuel their long-distance run. They were also able to use more fat oxidation at higher levels of intense activity that approached, but did not reach, anaerobic exercise. Keto athletes achieved approximately 70 percent of maximal oxygen carrying capacity, compared to only 55 percent in the athletes on high-carb diets. Interestingly, although some of the high-carb dieters in the study were able to increase their levels of ketones briefly during intense activity, their levels dropped significantly when they stopped exercise, while keto runners maintained ketosis throughout the day and only went deeper into ketosis during training.

A recent report of an endurance athlete highlights this. The athlete followed a keto lifestyle but decided to carb up before his workouts. He routinely ate 80 grams of daily carbs to fuel his high level of activity, but then added 60 grams of extra carbs pre-workout. During both his short sprint activities and his prolonged endurance activities, he noticed a decrease (albeit small at about 1.1 percent to 1.6 percent) in his performance. Yet, there was an increase of 2.8 percent in his high-intensity endurance exercise. His findings echo other studies.

In the highly trained athlete, keto:

>> Maintains — or even improves — endurance and sprint type activities

>> Decreases gains in high-intensity anaerobic-type activities

On keto, the human body is very capable of making all the glucose you need via gluconeogenesis, without having to rely on fattening and insulin-spiking carbs.

The body can ramp up ketone production during periods of exercise; some studies have shown that fat-adapted athletes triple their ketone production during medium- to high-intensity workouts. These findings suggest that being a keto-adapted athlete may result in lower systemic inflammation than is found in highly active athletes who stick to a carb-heavy diet.

Exercising while intermittent fasting

There are two camps of people:

>> **Those who feel that you must have some carbs actively being digested in your system to fuel up and make the most of your workout:** These folks refer to the thermic effect of exercise. Because food increases metabolism, the theory goes that by eating before your workout you prime your body to

be even more metabolically active. Also, many studies show that carbohydrates are preferentially used when your muscles are hard at work, making people think that this means that carbs are the best fuel for moving muscles.

>> **Those who swear by fasted workouts:** These folks suggest that the increase in ketones with an overnight fast will increase your body's ability to focus on fat oxidation. When stored fat and ketones are used to fuel your workout, you're likely to go straight to fat-burning mode rather than use your pre-workout shake to power your workout. If you're burning fat you already have, the theory goes, you're more likely to lose excess pounds. Also, the effect of fasting helps to produce more human growth hormone (HGH), which helps increase muscle gains over the long run.

The reality is that there is truth to both of these philosophies. What works best for an individual keto dieter depends on what she wants to gain from her exercise routine and what she is most comfortable with.

A recent meta-analysis of fasting or feeding on endurance training tried to settle the score. A meta-analysis allows researchers to combine the findings from multiple studies in hopes of finding a more balanced and accurate result. The study found no difference between the two groups. The meta-analysis showed

>> No significant difference in total body weight loss by either eating or fasting before a workout

>> No significant difference in total body fat loss between the two groups

TIP

You can rest assured that you're not putting yourself at a disadvantage by working out after an overnight fast.

REMEMBER

These individuals were not keto-adapted, meaning their results would be lower than the keto dieter who chooses to add intermittent fasting to the mix.

These studies were looking at fasted exercise in people who were doing primarily endurance-type activities, in which they were using about 60 percent to 65 percent of the oxygen-carrying capacity. So, what happens if you're doing another type of exercise?

Another study looked at NCAA Division 1 trained athletes who were asked to perform resistance-type training in both fasted and non-fasted states. Study participants were given a high-carb meal with approximately 50 grams of carbs on their non-fasted days, which is considered the typical "carb loading" that many targeted keto dieters use for fuel. The meal had only a small amount of protein (3.3 grams). In the study, participants performed the bench press, back squat, and military press at 60 percent of their personal bests. The results showed:

>> No difference between MET expended when fasting versus non-fasting

>> No difference between heart rate or athlete's perceived exertion during fasting versus non-fasting

>> An increase in fat oxidation (metabolism) in the fasted state compared to the non-fasted state

TIP

Studies have repeatedly failed to find any significant difference between working out in a fasted or non-fasted state. These terms generally apply to those who are fasting for less than 24 hours — if you're fasting for longer than that, you shouldn't be engaging in strenuous exercise. A fasted state essentially means that you haven't eaten your first meal of the day before you exercise. Just make sure that you eat immediately following a workout, because that's when your muscles need it the most.

Adjusting Your Macros to Accommodate Exercise

Regardless of which type of exercise you do, you need make your nutrients work for you to reach your fitness goals. In this section, we look at three goals — muscle gains, fat loss, and building endurance — and tell you the best way to meet them.

Optimizing muscle gain

When exercising on the keto diet, protein (not fat) is paramount. Some highly trained athletes on keto chose to do a protein-rich keto diet where their protein accounts for 35 percent rather than 20 percent of total caloric intake. Why is this important?

>> Protein improves satiety, meaning you're less likely to stuff your face after a workout and fall behind on your weight loss goals.

>> Protein enhances muscle cell growth, which is torn down by exercise and in a recovery period for several hours after you finish working out.

>> Protein is more metabolically active than other macronutrients, meaning that it will help burn fat more quickly.

>> Protein is necessary for muscle recovery and maintenance.

The ratio of protein you need depends on your activity level. The recommended daily allowance (RDA) for protein for most healthy individuals is 0.36 gram per pound per day. However, that takes into account a wide range of adults from the sedentary office worker to elite bodybuilders. Obviously, this won't work for everyone. The International Society of Sports Nutrition (ISSN) laid out a better option for active individuals:

>> **Endurance athletes (for example, long-distance runner, cyclists, and swimmers):** 0.45 to 0.72 gram per pound per day

>> **Intermittent-style activities athletes (those who don't fall into the other two categories, including many kinds of athletes and those who combine endurance-type training with intermittent explosive force):** 0.63 to 0.77 gram per pound per day

>> **Resistance/weight-training athletes (for example, bodybuilders and powerlifters):** 0.72 to 0.9 gram per pound per day and occasionally even more than 1.36 grams per pound per day for high-intensity athletes who want to lose weight

TIP

So, when should you take your protein? Throughout the day, but "protein load" around the time that you plan to exercise. Studies show a benefit of protein intake before, during, and after exercise, so whichever works best for you is what you should choose.

Post-exercise protein

Your body is primed to build muscle in the 24 hours after you've done a hard bout of resistance-type exercise. Protein ingested within 30 minutes of completing your exercise routine will provide the amino acids you need for continued muscle growth. Protein ingestion after a workout tells your muscle cells to grow larger. This leads to an overall increase in muscle protein synthesis (MPS).

Timing your protein intake within 30 minutes of the end of your workout provides the most substantial amount of muscle growth stimulation (for both aerobic and anaerobic exercise). This is because

>> The initiation of muscle growth typically occurs within 30 to 60 minutes after a workout.

>> Protein intake within two hours of a workout improves signaling pathways that increase muscle fiber growth, as well as replenishing glycogen stores.

>> Post-workout MPS peaks within three hours of exercise and remains elevated for a day or longer.

The ISSN recommends a goal of eating about 20 to 40 grams of protein around the time of your workout.

Endurance athletes (for example, very long-distance runners or triathletes) who require nutrition during exercise should consume 0.11 gram of protein per pound per hour to decrease muscle strain. Generally, you'll need to be exercising for at least 60 minutes to require this. The benefit is that it minimizes muscle damage and aids muscle recovery. Most people don't need to ingest protein as they're exercising if there is a lot of downtime between exercises.

TIP

With all that said, the timing of your protein intake is less important than making sure you're getting enough protein for your exercise routine. Make sure you're getting around 0.68 gram per pound of protein per day if you're active and want to build muscle. You may need more if you're doing resistance-type training. If you're trying to increase your lean muscle mass, you'll need enough protein to not only maintain, but also build, your muscle.

Specific types of protein to improve muscle gains

Essential amino acids (EAAs) deserve a special mention when we discuss protein and muscle growth. The EEAs are

>> Histidine

>> Isoleucine

>> Leucine

>> Lysine

>> Methionine

>> Phenylalanine

>> Threonine

>> Tryptophan

>> Valine

These are building blocks for all the muscles in your body. The human body is unable to make these amino acids, so we have to get them from either the foods we eat or as supplements. EAAs are the most critical stimulators for MPS, which puts athletes in a positive nitrogen balance (or muscle-building state).

We also should talk a little bit about a subgroup of the EEA, called the branch-chained amino acids (BCAAs):

>> Leucine

>> Isoleucine

>> Valine

These three amino acids account for about a third of the muscle in the body, but more important, they play a significant role in making muscle and assisting in its recovery. They tend to be more efficient because the liver can transport them directly to the muscle without having to undergo a more complex pathway to be metabolized. Studies show that these amino acids help to increase the amount of protein you make and decrease the amount you lose. That's a win-win for anyone who is trying to sculpt a leaner physique. Studies show that these combinations are beneficial both for endurance-type exercise, as well as resistance training.

In moderate long-distance activity, BCAAs helped to

>> Improve the performance of long-distance runners

>> Decrease the subjective feeling of fatigue

Some research even suggests that BCAAs are essential for boosting your brain power. Generally, the goal is to consume more than 20 milligrams per pound per day of leucine and more than 10 milligrams per pound per day of both isoleucine and valine, since this is the natural ratio (2:1:1) that BCAAs appear in most animal protein. The ISSN suggest that you should have a goal of eating 700 to 3,000 milligrams of leucine at any one time and eat these regularly throughout the day.

BCAAs are found in all protein-rich foods, but they're highest in red meats and dairy, like the following:

>> Beef

>> Goat

>> Lamb

>> Hard cheeses

>> Whey (in low-carb protein powders)

REMEMBER

It's best to get these amino acids from whole-food sources, so don't feel compelled to go out and buy EAA or BCAA supplements. Instead, stick to a diet that has all the amino acids you need and choose a protein powder (we include a breakdown of the details you need to know later in this chapter) that is well-rounded if you want to build mass. Studies show that people who take protein powder, rather than merely a specific list of amino acids, do better in terms of stimulating their muscle growth potential.

WARNING

There is a point at which too much protein becomes a detriment for the keto athlete. For keto athletes, excess protein does turn into glucose via gluconeogenesis, so it's best to take in the protein you need and not overdo it, even around of the time of your workout. You don't want to increase the risk that you'll get knocked out of ketosis.

REMEMBER

The amount of protein you take in depends on your goals. Factor in the type of activity you usually do, any changes in weight goals, and how much muscle or endurance you want to build.

Optimizing fat loss

If your goal is to lose fat, you have to make changes to both your diet and your exercise routine. Figuring out your optimal protein intake is essential to losing weight. Make sure to really dig into the preceding section to get the whole picture on how building lean muscle will aid in your fat loss.

Next, you need to evaluate your fat intake to reach your goals. On the keto diet, fat can range from 65 percent to 85 percent of your total caloric intake, so there is a range to choose from to reach your optimal lean body mass. For fat loss, your goal should be about 65 percent to 70 percent of your total intake. When you cut calories to achieve your goal, the calories should come from your fat intake.

REMEMBER

A pound of weight is about 3,500 calories, so to lose half a pound to a pound a week, you'll need to shave off 250 to 500 calories per day (whether through diet or exercise, or a combination of both).

WARNING

Refrain from trying to lose fat too quickly; it's often unsustainable to slash calories by more than 500 calories per day over the long term because you'll just end up feeling sluggish and hungry. Besides, you risk losing some of the hard-earned muscle you've built.

Adjusting for endurance

Many keto-adapted athletes are able to maintain keto without losing performance. If you're a bodybuilder or long-distance runner, you have a distinct advantage because your muscles will naturally turn to fat for energy when carb-heavy athletes use glucose. In fact, many of the studies that look at endurance athletes show performance at moderate activity levels (an average of about 60 percent of maximal aerobic power) peaked on keto. That's because they were burning more fat — a more plentiful source of energy — earlier and longer than athletes who primarily used glycogen or glucose instead, which has a limited supply.

Because you'll be burning more fat throughout all parts of your workout as an endurance athlete, you likely won't notice any changes in your performance. It's important to remember, however, that this won't happen immediately, and during your transition, you may see more fatigue and muscle soreness as your body turns from using glucose to leveraging fat for fuel.

TIP

Generally, it's a good idea to stay on the standard ketogenic diet with carbohydrates levels of 20 to 50 grams per day and see how you do on your exercise regimen. Give it a solid two weeks before making any changes.

On the other hand, if you do intermittent-style activities — tennis, basketball, and others — that require short but high-intensity bursts of action over and over again, you may notice some dips in your performance. That's because these high-intensity moves need glucose for fuel. With a low-carb diet, your muscles just won't have enough carbs to fuel high-intensity actions (around 80 percent or more of your max capacity) for longer than 10 seconds. If you primarily engage in one of these sports, then it's best to try some carbs around the time of your exercise to boost your glucose utilization.

WARNING

There is little benefit to adding carbs after, as opposed to before, your workout. Studies show that it's protein intake *after* the exercise that is important and carbs are primarily beneficial for glycogen replenishment.

Choosing the Right Style of Keto for Your Unique Goals

In Chapter 1, we touch upon the different forms of keto available. Here we explain why you might choose one of these styles, based on your exercise routine, to make the most of keto.

Following the standard ketogenic diet

For the vast majority of keto dieters, the standard option is the best. Although it has been drilled into our heads that carbs are necessary for muscle function and performance, the truth is that you can still be very active without having to eat excess carbs to fuel your workouts. The vast majority of us are not Olympic level body lifters or CrossFit Athletes, and the minor drops in performance probably are made up by the health benefits of going keto. Also, the standard keto diet is quite adequate for most activities done on a recreational basis, including endurance and resistance type activities.

TIP

Stick with a standard keto diet if any of the following apply to you:

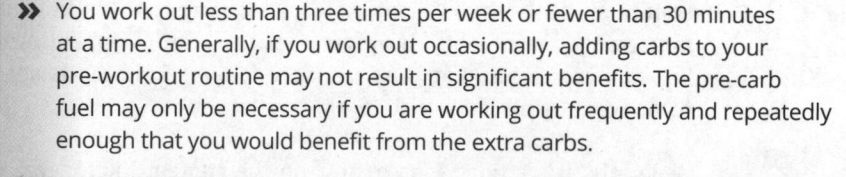

>> You work out less than three times per week or fewer than 30 minutes at a time. Generally, if you work out occasionally, adding carbs to your pre-workout routine may not result in significant benefits. The pre-carb fuel may only be necessary if you are working out frequently and repeatedly enough that you would benefit from the extra carbs.

>> You primarily do aerobic or endurance-style activities that are moderate in intensity. These types of activities are the ones that thrive on ketones. If you are keto-adapted, you shouldn't notice a drop in your performance.

>> You've experiences significant health benefits from going keto, like improvement in blood pressure or diabetes.

>> You haven't really noticed any change in your performance. If your performance level is stable, don't increase your carb count.

If your goal is to lose fat or even maintain your weight and you primarily walk, run, or do low amounts of HIIT or light resistance training, then standard keto is the best option and will provide enough energy to fuel your workout and allow you to achieve your health goals.

Following a high-protein ketogenic diet to build muscle mass

Most high-intensity resistance athletes who do keto will choose the high-protein diet to fall into line with what the ISSN recommends for protein intake. Remember that the ISSN suggests that you need to eat a significant amount of protein— between 0.72 to 0.9 gram per pound per day — to build muscle while lifting heavy. This amount of protein all but requires that you choose the high-protein keto diet, where protein makes up as much as 30 percent of your total caloric intake.

If you go as high a 1.36 grams per pound of protein or more, you will be eating a high-protein keto diet, and you'll need to adjust the other levels of your caloric intake to compensate.

Regardless, there are some negatives to overeating protein:

>> Protein stimulates insulin production. While insulin has some muscle building benefits during your workout, too much insulin can negate the benefits of keto.

>> Excess protein can kick-start gluconeogenesis. If you overdo it on protein, the excess may go toward making glucose. You will notice fewer ketones as you increase your protein intake and may even get kicked out of ketosis if you consume significantly more than your level of exercise requires.

REMEMBER

A high-protein keto diet is a good option for those who want to build muscle mass and focus primarily on resistance-style training. It's unlikely to kick you out of ketosis unless you increase your protein higher than the recommended 30 percent of total calories.

Following a targeted ketogenic diet to build workout progress

If you're doing primarily CrossFit workouts or strength training, it may be useful to choose the targeted version of the keto diet. In this regimen, you'd eat 20 to 50 grams of fast-acting carbs around half an hour to an hour before your workout. This would be in addition to the carbs you generally consume with the standard keto diet.

The reasoning behind this is that you'll have quick-acting glucose to power your muscle for the maximum, all-out exercise you need. Even as a keto-adapted athlete, you need some glucose or glycogen to fuel your anaerobic exercise.

If you want to lose weight, calculate the extra calories from the extra 20 to 50 grams of pre-workout carbs, and subtract that from your total caloric intake. Start with 20 grams and then tailor to your needs. That means that on the days that you work out, you'll be eating a little less fat than on non-workout days.

TIP

Consider a targeted keto diet if any of the following applies to you:

>> **You won't have to kick yourself out of ketosis for long periods to be able to make gains on HIIT and weight lifting.** This is preferential for people who have metabolic reasons for staying away from carbs (like diabetes) and don't want to go back to the ups and downs of a high-carb lifestyle.

>> **It decreases your perceived effort of doing the same activity if you have carbs.** As we mention earlier, endurance athletes who ate carbs before their workout felt like it was easier to finish their race, making workouts more pleasurable and sustainable.

>> **It may boost some muscle gains during your workout because the added carbs will increase insulin.** In this one case — right before a workout — insulin isn't as bad because it drives amino acids into muscle cells, fueling your body's repair efforts.

Targeted keto may be for you if you're noticing consistent decreases in your performance and you feel like you always hit a wall during your workouts. Basically, the targeted keto diet is best for athletes who have noticed a drop in their results since going keto. Alternatively, targeted keto may be useful for some elite endurance athletes who, although keto-adapted, are still noticing that they aren't hitting their personal bests in long-distance activities.

TIP

Before your workout, choose fast-acting carbs that will be able to power you through your workout. Avoid eating junk food that can leave you feeling sluggish before your workout, so stick to healthier forms of carbs if you choose the targeted keto route.

TIP

You can add some protein to your pre-workout carbs — this may provide an additional energy boost — but stay away from high-fat foods because they'll slow down the absorption of your carbs. The only fats you should consider consuming immediately before your workout are medium-chain triglyceride (MCT) oils, which are very fast absorbing and help increase your ketones. Pre-workout ketones not only help fuel your muscles but may help prevent you from being kicked out of ketosis with the excess carbs you're eating.

Using a cyclical ketogenic diet for your endurance goals

The cyclical keto diet is for the competitive strength-training athlete who just needs more carbs for high-level anaerobic exercise. Not many people fall into this category, so odds are, this section doesn't apply to you.

WILL A TARGETED KETO DIET KICK ME OUT OF KETOSIS?

The honest answer is that it depends. Everyone is different, and it'll take some trial and error to make sure targeted keto works for you. Not everyone on keto is limited to the same number of carbs, and every workout is different. Your ketosis depends on a few key factors:

- Your sensitivity to carbs (how insulin sensitive you are)
- Whether you're keto-adapted (which indicates how well your body burns ketones for fuel)
- How many carbs (and the type) you eat before your workout
- The length and intensity of your workout

It's critical to determine how you feel after working out with extra carbs. If you notice improve performance and energy at 20 grams of carbs, there is no need to eat any more. However, if it takes more carbs to get to the same level of performance, you may be at higher risk of being kicked out of ketosis.

Some people choose to check their ketones after their workouts to see if they're in ketosis and adapt based on the results. This approach is probably only useful if you're noticing side effects from adding carbs and you think that you've been kicked out of ketosis. It can give you insight to determine if you can increase or decrease the amount of carbs you consume before exercising.

Of course, everyone who consumes carbs will notice a drop in the level of ketones immediately afterward, so don't let this alarm you. As long as you keep the carbs to a pre-workout routine, your muscles will consume the majority of the carbs so that your body will be back to exclusively burning ketones soon after your workout is over.

If this is all too confusing, it may be helpful to seek out a knowledgeable keto nutritionist or personal trainer to help you figure out the right level of carbs pre-workout for you based on your unique situation.

Remember: You should be keto-adapted before you switch to a targeted keto diet. This means that you should have been following keto for at least two months or longer and have stable ketone levels before you start adding excess carbs before your workout.

TIP

Consider the cyclical keto diet if any of the following applies to you:

>> **You are an elite bodybuilder or short-distance sprinter who has been training for years.** And you've noticed drops in your performance and realize that you need more carbs to fuel your intense level of activity.

>> **You are otherwise healthy and don't have any metabolic reasons that carb loading will affect your health.** If you noticed an improvement in blood pressure or blood sugar levels, cyclical keto is *not* for you, because you may lose all your gains when you cycle out of ketosis.

>> **You work out intensely and on a specific schedule.** Your high-carb days should coincide with the days that you're at the gym. Also, you'll need to be able to cycle in and out of ketosis by completely depleting the excess carbs you consume on your workout days and then switch back into a keto diet on non-carb-loading days.

Generally, cyclical keto will help with gains in the anaerobic type of exercise. That means 100-meter sprints, low-rep maximums (five or six) for weight lifters, or for CrossFit circuits.

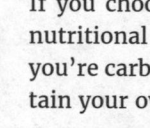

REMEMBER

If you choose the cyclical keto diet, you still have to keep an eye on your total nutritional needs and don't forget about your total caloric intake on the days that you're carb loading. You'll need to drop your fat intake on your carb days to maintain your overall caloric needs.

TIP

Most people go back to a standard American diet ratio of macronutrients on a carb day. That means getting about 60 percent to 70 percent of your calories from carbs, 20 percent to 25 percent from protein, and only 10 percent or less from fat.

Unlike the targeted keto diet, you're going to be eating complex carbohydrates on your carb days. These carbs will help you replenish the glycogen stores in your muscle cells and will be less likely to cause intense spikes in your insulin levels like highly refined carbs would. You need to make sure you're eating nutrient-dense carbs on this diet.

Carbs to eat on the cyclical diet include

>> Sweet potatoes

>> Squash

>> Quinoa

>> Beans or lentils

>> Whole grains

Although high in carbs, these foods are more nutrient-dense than quick-absorbing carbs and tend to pack in the right amount of minerals, vitamins, and fiber for overall health.

There are some downsides to the cyclical keto diet:

>> **It's a bit more difficult to cycle in and out of ketosis, and some people struggle, feeling as though they're always chasing and checking their ketone levels.** On the days of carb loading, you'll push your body completely out of ketosis, and it may be difficult to jump right back into ketosis on your keto days, even if you go back to a standard keto diet. Its why it's essential that on the cyclical keto diet — even more so than the other forms — you're entirely keto adapted before you transition to this more advanced form of dieting.

Some people find they need to be even stricter on keto days, sticking to 20 grams of carbs or less to get back in ketosis. Other people find that they need to add in intermittent fasting in between cyclical and standard keto days. Some find that this is a great time to do a fasted workout. People on the cyclical diet may find that it takes a while to get into a balance of cycling back and forth between ketosis and carb loading.

>> **Adding carbs back into your diet on refeeding days may lead to yo-yo weight changes because you'll add back a lot of water weight on carb refeed days.** You may also find that it's more difficult to lose weight — and you may even gain fat — on the keto diet because many people find it easy to overconsume calories on their refeeding days. Carbs aren't as filling as fat is, so you'll soon learn that you won't feel as satiated with the same number of calories on carb days as you do on keto days.

There isn't enough research on the cyclical diet to know its pros and cons, although a couple of studies have looked at this. One study examined elite race walkers who were split equally among three dietary options: a standard American diet high in carbs, a keto-style diet with 75 percent to 80 percent of calories from fat, and a blended diet in which the standard American diet was mixed with intermittent fasting and low carb availability. The keto dieters showed improved fat oxidation, but worse performance after three weeks on the diet, while the blended dieters (similar to the high-carb group) showed an improvement in performance of the study test.

Because the research is so limited, we do have to rely primarily on anecdotal advice and what we've personally noticed from people who choose to do the cyclical diet. The metabolic effects of cycling in and out of ketosis are unknown. It may not be as helpful in maintaining the health benefits of ketosis, such as lower blood pressure and increased insulin sensitivity, because you're actively consuming excess carbs on certain days. Still, even on the cyclical diet, you're eating fewer carbs than on the standard American diet, so it does make sense that you'll see some benefits of ketosis, even if they aren't as high as on the standard keto diet.

REMEMBER

A cyclical keto diet is only an option for athletes who work out at intense levels regularly. There isn't much research on cyclical keto, so you may need to do some fine-tuning. Also, you may not get all the health benefits of keto when you cycle in and out of ketosis regularly.

Adapting Your Exercise Routine

Recommendations from the American Heart Association (AHA) and the American College of Sports Medicine (ACSM) suggest that adults need to get at least 150 to 250 minutes of exercise per week to avoid gaining weight, and more than 250 minutes per week for significant weight loss. Also, the AHA recommends "muscle strengthening" activities two times per week. The traditional recommendations encourage people to get most of this exercise as moderate aerobic activity (or endurance training); they can cut the amount of time in half by increasing the effort to a vigorous level (a MET of 8 or more).

Newer research is looking to see if these recommendations are sound for everyone's health and fitness goals. Generally speaking, however, we need to do a range of physical activities to stay our healthiest. Goals differ from person to person, but exercise on the keto diet can help achieve all of the following:

>> Losing weight

>> Building muscle

>> Treating or preventing diseases like diabetes, high blood pressure, and cancer

>> Improving mental health

>> Living longer

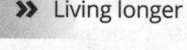

TIP

The first thing you need to identify is your goals: What do you want to achieve by exercising on keto? When you know what your goal is, then you can choose the activities and the eating style that will help you accomplish that goal. In this section, we cover the types of exercises you should consider.

Anaerobic exercise: High-intensity interval training and resistance training

Resistance or strength training is any form of movement in which your body and your muscles have to move against a force opposing your muscles. Most people think of weight lifting as the quintessential resistance training, but there are many more, such as:

>> Body-weight exercises like push-ups and pull-ups

>> Dragging sleds

>> Running with resistance (such as a weighted vest)

>> Water aerobics

HITT is another form of anaerobic exercise that pushes your muscles to their limit. As it has increased in popularity, more and more people are using HIIT with the thought that it will improve fat loss in a shorter time than more traditional forms of exercise. Studies show that doing HIIT for half the time as regular aerobic or cardiovascular activity seems to increase weight and fat loss.

TIP

If you're interested in HIIT, but you're not sure where to get started, try some of the workouts at www.dummies.com/health/exercise/weights/the-basics-of-high-intensity-interval-training/, or search the web for "HIIT videos" to find some videos you can work out with.

The selling points of these two types of exercise are that not only do they build muscles, but they do so better than any other form of exercise while still helping you lose weight. Because muscle is more metabolically active than any other part of your body, people who build muscle have a higher baseline metabolism than someone of the same weight who has less muscle mass.

Studies show that increasing muscle mass from weight lifting increased resting metabolism by 4 percent in women and almost 10 percent in healthy young men. Research also indicates that strength training is vital for improving insulin sensitivity, and it's an excellent way to maintain bone integrity, a common concern as people age. Overall, resistance training improves body fat percentage by increasing lean muscle mass.

Aerobic exercise

Aerobic exercise is probably what you think of when you think of exercise. Anything that gets your heart rate up by making your cardiovascular system work harder is aerobic exercise. It's the exercise that relies on the body's use of oxygen — as compared to short, intense bouts of exercise that depend on fast-acting creatine phosphate or on anaerobic metabolism.

During cardiovascular exercise, the heart gets a great workout, and you're able to sustain the level of activity for more extended periods than with anaerobic exercise. There is a wide range of aerobic exercise that goes from mild to vigorous, but you should aim for a level of activity you can continue for a more extended period to truly call it endurance.

Common forms of aerobic exercise include

>> Aerobic-style classes like Zumba

>> Running

>> Brisk walking

>> Cycling

>> Swimming

>> Cross-country skiing

>> Jumping rope

Aerobic-style exercise is the best option if you're looking to drop calories quickly. This form of movement tends to burn more calories than resistance training — it can even be as high as two times as many calories burned compared to weight training in the same amount of time. Yet, you're less likely to pack on as much metabolically active muscle as you would with weight training, meaning that your resting metabolism may not improve as much. Aerobic exercise decreases your percent body fat by reducing overall fat mass.

Aerobic exercise has been studied extensively and is the form of training with the most known benefits. It's a phenomenal workout for the heart, and it has been proven to decrease the risk of cardiovascular diseases like stroke and heart attacks, while also being beneficial at reducing rates of diabetes and high blood pressure.

Balance or stability

Although less commonly thought of as exercise, balance or stability movements also deserve mention. Many other types of exercise include balance, but the AHA defines these movements as necessary for increasing functional activities and building strength and confidence. They're especially important for older people to decrease their risks of falls.

Because these movements are slow and don't use a lot of weight, they're often considered a mild form of exercise, and you'd be hard pressed to lose a lot of weight committing only to these kinds of activity unless you're cutting way down on calories. However, if you incorporate these type of movements into strength-based activities and cardio exercises, you can increase their metabolic effect.

Balance and stability movements often focus on core body movements so you may notice a tighter and more centered *core* (abdominal and back muscles).

Some common movements that incorporate balance–style exercise include

>> **T'ai chi:** T'ai chi is a Chinese martial art system that consists of sequences of slow, controlled movements. If you've ever seen a friend or an actor on the silver screen doing a rehearsed sequence as a form of meditation, it was either t'ai chi or a very similar art. Check out *T'ai Chi For Dummies,* by Therese Iknoian (Wiley) to learn more about this form of exercise.

>> **Exercise using BOSU balls:** BOSU balls are very popular not only in the gym, but also in physical therapy offices. They look like someone cut the top third off of an exercise ball and attached it to a flat plastic base. BOSU balls offer a wide range of bodyweight strengthening activities, allowing you to exercise your core while doing a number of simple exercises such as push-ups, sit-ups, squats, and lunges.

>> **Curtsy lunges:** This variation of the lunge targets the inner thighs and several buttocks muscles. To do a curtsy lunge, stand in a normal squat position; then step forward with your right foot and cross it in front of your left foot while kneeling. Stand back up and repeat on the opposite side.

>> **Weight shifts:** This exercise is often targeted at older individuals to keep them in shape and well balanced, but it can also be an excellent warm-up or cooldown exercise for all ages. To do them, simply engage in exaggerated forms of typical movements, such as swaying side to side and taking larger than normal steps. Dealing with these exaggerated movements keeps you well balanced.

>> **Pistol squats:** Not for the faint of heart, and certainly the most advanced exercise on this list. To do a pistol squat, you lift one leg and stretch it out in front of you while trying to grab it with one hand; at the same time, you squat and support your entire body weight on the other leg. Stand and repeat the exercise on the opposite side. This is a worthy goal — if you can do pistol squats, you're almost certainly in excellent shape!

Flexibility or stretching

Flexibility and stretching are usually part of the warm–up routine, but they're benefits are likely more significant if you incorporate them *after* you exercise. Some studies have shown as much as a 17 percent increase in muscle mass gained by athletes who stretch immediately following a training session.

Stretching is a valuable part of training. It can warm up your muscles and is often invaluable in decreasing your risk of sprains and injuries after you do any other type of exercise. Flexibility also improves posture and balance and can enhance your range of motion for both strength and aerobic activities. Like balance movement, flexibility exercise can be incorporated into aerobic or strength-training activities to improve their effectiveness.

Some common flexibility activities include:

>> **Yoga:** This exercise system focuses on holding poses that slightly stretch you for long periods of time. Yoga uses breath control, specific body postures, and simple meditation. Check out *Yoga For Dummies,* 3rd Edition, by Larry Payne and Georg Feuerstein (Wiley), for more information.

>> **Dynamic stretches:** These stretches are done using body movement to create a slight stretch with each repetition. Examples include twisting side to side to stretch your core and swinging your arms back and forth to warm up or cool down your arm, chest, and upper-back muscles. Focus on dynamic stretches when warming up.

>> **Static stretches:** These stretches use positions that are held in place for a certain period of time. Yoga employs a full workout routine, but static stretching is typically an ad-hoc activity, focused on where your body needs it and only done for a few minutes. Static stretches are most useful for cooldowns.

MIXING AND MATCHING

Many people incorporate bits and pieces of each style of exercise into a single fitness routine. There is no reason why you can't mix your flexibility training with resistance or incorporate aerobic and anaerobic forms of exercise at the same time.

In fact, it's probably best to do *all* forms of exercise to get a range of benefits. Studies that looked at individuals who were committed to both aerobic and resistance training noted that they lost more weight and gained more muscle than individuals who spent the same time doing just one form of exercise.

In one study, the group pursuing a resistance training program didn't lose as much weight as those in the aerobic group, who did the equivalent of running 12 miles per week. However, those who *combined* the activities, although they spent longer working out, saw an increase in both fat loss *and* muscle gains.

Bonus workouts to reach your goals

We've got you covered if you'd like some easy-to-follow workout routines attuned to your personal goals. Here are two of our favorites.

Fat loss routine

Aerobic exercise is the best way to burn fat immediately, but it requires that you put some significant work in and occasionally go to your max capacity. If you're consuming enough calories and protein, this will not detract from your benefit, even on keto.

Anaerobic exercise is where you push beyond your limits, finding the sweet point between lactate buildup and making muscle gains. Because muscle is the most metabolically active part of your body, it will help you continue to burn fat even after your workout is done. This is the beauty of HIIT and why you should aim for high intensity followed by moderate intensity workouts for your fat loss routine.

Do this circuit twice while maintaining good form. It should take 12 minutes in total.

1. **For 40 seconds, do side lunges.**

Stand with your feet shoulder-width apart, and then step out to the right side with your right leg while bending down in a lunging movement. Return to standing, and then repeat on the other side.

2. **For 20 seconds, jump rope or do high knees.**

Run in place, lifting your knees as high as you can.

3. **For 40 seconds, do burpees.**

Begin in the standing position, and then bend over at the waist and place your hands on the ground in front of your feet (you'll likely have to bend your knees to do this). Step back with both feet until you're in the push-up position. Complete one push-up, and then bring your legs back up to their original positions, and stand back up. That whole movement counts as one burpee.

4. **For 20 seconds, jump rope or do knee highs.**

5. **For 40 seconds, do standard lunges or jump lunges.**

If you're a beginner, do standard lunges: Stand with your feet shoulder-width apart, and then step forward with one foot and kneel down until your knee nearly touches the floor. Ideally, each of your legs will form a 90-degree angle in the down position. Alternate legs.

If you're advanced, consider doing a jump squat: Begin by standing with your feet shoulder-width apart; then make a small jump in the air and bring your legs into the lunge position, dropping rapidly to the ground. Jump back up and switch legs — if your right leg was in front the first time, put your left leg out first the second.

6. **For 20 seconds, jump rope or do knee highs.**

7. **For 40 seconds, do regular squats or pistol squats.**

   A pistol squat is an advanced technique: Lift one leg and stretch it out in front while trying to grab it with one hand, while you squat and support your entire body weight on the other leg. Stand and repeat the exercise on the opposite side.

   Until you're ready for this, do standard squats.

8. **For 20 seconds, jump rope or do knee highs.**

9. **For 40 seconds, do a side curtsy.**

   This movement begins with a standard side lunge. As you're coming back up, take the same leg that went out to the side and extend it behind you and to the opposite side, kneeling down as if you were curtsying. For example, you would extend your right leg out to the side, kneel, and then as you stand back up, extend your right leg back and to the left side, kneeling in a curtsy. Return to a standing position and repeat on the other side.

10. **For 20 seconds, jump rope or do knee highs.**

11. **For 40 seconds, do high planks to forearm planks.**

    High planks are essentially the up push-up position: Your hands and toes are the only things touching the ground and your arms are fully extended. Forearm planks are the same basic position, but they involve resting on your elbows and forearms instead of your hands.

    To complete this exercise, begin in the high planks position, and then go down to the forearm planks position one arm at a time. To complete one repetition, return to the high planks position using only your arms (don't let your knees touch the floor).

12. **For 20 seconds, jump rope or do knee highs.**

You should be pretty breathless during and after this routine. Remember to keep good form as a priority, even if you have to slow down your repetitions to maintain it.

If you want to understand what a basic movement looks like, go to YouTube and search for that particular exercise. You'll find dozens of form videos for every movement. If you feel unsure or unsafe, we always recommend finding a personal trainer to help you learn new techniques or movements.

Endurance routine

Endurance means giving your cardiovascular system a workout and making it more efficient so you can go faster, longer, or harder. This is not the same as fat loss — you can increase your endurance while gaining weight. Ever notice that you can gain weight even though you can run farther? That's because your body has decreased the amount of energy to do the same work — your metabolism has slowed down so that the same work requires less effort on your body's part.

If your goal is to get better at something, this isn't a bad thing, but it's important to be aware that endurance does that — it makes you better, but not necessarily thinner. You can increase your endurance levels by alternating between light and moderate intensity. (Think about the difference between exercising at a level you can sustain for several hours, and then increasing it to a high-exertion activity for a minute or less, and then going back down.) Generally, endurance requires a longer time commitment compared to fat loss.

The key to endurance is to reduce the amount of rest between reps to help build stamina. You'll also need to know your one-repetition maximum and shoot for about 50 percent of that for about three sets of 10 to 25 reps each. Your one-rep max is the amount you can safely lift or move during a single repetition. Don't attempt a one-rep maximum until you have been working out for a few months and are familiar with proper form and have a good idea of what your body can do. To build endurance, you'll want to shorten your rest periods between sets to less than 90 seconds.

Here are some of the major cornerstone exercises you'll employ in a gym. Because these involve free weights, form is an absolute must. If you don't know how to do these safely, ask a trainer for help:

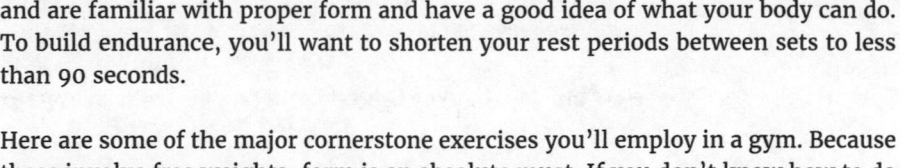

>> **Weighted squats:** These use the same basic form as a standard squat, but hold a barbell across your shoulders with weight on it.

>> **Deadlifts:** Place a barbell with on the floor. Stand behind the barbell, place your hands slightly wider than shoulder-width apart, and slowly stand up to lift the barbell; then return it to the ground.

>> **Bench press:** Lie on your back on a bench, and press a barbell to the sky with your arms as it lies across your chest.

>> **Rows:** Rows involve any kind of pulling motion that simulates the basic rowing motion you would do in a boat. Variations of this activity put your body in various positions and orientations to work your back muscles differently.

With this endurance training routine, you should feel your heart rate increase. An added bonus is that this may also help to accentuate your muscle-building efforts so you'll notice an improvement in metabolism.

Considering Supplements That May Help

When you combine keto and exercise, you're adding two great options to help you achieve your fitness goals, whatever they may be. Most people get the vast majority of the benefits from these two endeavors without any supplements. Still, there are some proven supplements that you may find useful depending on your goals.

Low-carb protein supplements

These are some of the best supplements for muscle gains. While you're on a keto diet, you should be able to get all your protein in a whole-food form, but sometimes you just need to supplement to make your macro goals. This may be especially true if you're increasing your percentage of protein intake to improve your muscle gains (for example, if you're on a high-protein keto diet). There are a lot of protein powders out there, but some are better suited for the keto diet.

There are two ways to classify protein powders:

>> **How quickly they're absorbed:** You can find the following types of protein powder:

- **Fast acting:** These protein powders are quickly digested and absorbed, so they're readily available for your muscles at your next workout.

- **Slow absorbing:** These protein powders take a while to be absorbed and digested, generally around six hours or longer. They aren't a useful fuel immediately before your workout, but they can help keep you satiated between meals and may help decrease muscle breakdown.

>> **How much protein is contained in the powder:** You have a few options:

- **Concentrates:** These protein powders include about 70 percent to 80 percent protein with the rest of the content coming from water, fats, carbs, and minerals.

- **Isolates:** These protein powders pack more protein, coming in at about 90 percent to 95 percent protein per weight, with even more non-protein components removed to increase their effectiveness.

- **Hydrolysates:** These protein powders have the proteins broken down into *peptides* and *polypeptides,* the smaller building blocks of protein. Although they aren't as tiny as amino acids, they make it that much easier for your body to absorb and digest the protein quickly. Because these protein powders are more quickly available, they can increase muscle by peaking insulin levels — and insulin's muscle-building effects — more.

In the following sections, we walk you through some types of protein powder you can choose among.

Whey protein

Whey protein is about 20 percent of the protein found in milk. This is a good go-to for a rapid-absorbing, well-rounded protein source. It has all the EAAs and BCAAs you need so you won't have to get these separately. In fact, it has the ideal BCAA ratio found in nature (2:1:1 of leucine to isoleucine and valine), making it a perfect protein. (See "Specific types of protein to improve muscle gains," earlier in this chapter, for more on EAAs and BCAAs.)

Whey is quickly digested by most people and taken up by your muscle cells for quick action. Its peak levels occur about an hour and a half after you take it. However, if you're lactose intolerant, whey concentrate is not the best option for you, and you should try either the isolate or a non–milk–based powder.

Here are some of the core benefits of whey protein:

>> **It's the best protein powder for encouraging muscle protein synthesis.** It stimulates proteins more than twice as much as casein protein. Studies show that taking 25 grams of fast-acting whey protein, rather than sipping it over the course of three hours, increases total MPS more. If increasing MPS during your workout is your goal, whey protein is a no-brainer. (See "Post-exercise protein," earlier in this chapter, for more on MPS.)

>> **It stimulates metabolism (meaning you burn more calories) more than most other types of protein powder.**

>> **It increases fat loss.** Research shows that people who supplemented with whey protein reduced fat around their midsections, the exact kind of fat that is associated with worse health outcomes.

Most people will aim to get 20 to 40 grams of protein about half an hour to an hour before a workout.

Casein protein

This is the main protein in milk. However, unlike whey, it's a slow-absorbing protein. It can take up to six hours for casein to be completely digested by your body, so it's not a good option just before your workouts. It doesn't boost MPS as much as whey protein does, but it may be more useful in limiting muscle break-down because it comes packed with glutamine, an amino acid that helps prevent muscle degeneration and also stimulates HGH. Overall, casein is still a good option for fat loss and muscle building in the long run.

Generally, casein protein should be taken in between meals or even right before bed. Some studies show that it can help minimize the natural muscle breakdown that happens as you sleep. You should aim for about 20 grams of casein between meals or at night if you choose to take it then.

Milk protein

Some people try to get the best of both worlds with milk protein, which has an 80:20 ratio of casein to whey so that you get the quick benefits of whey and the extended and slow release of protein from casein. It has all your required EAAs and BCAAS, making it a great option. Milk protein is often found in some protein bars and protein powder blend.

Egg protein

For those of us who are allergic to milk products, egg protein is another valid option. It's primarily made from egg whites, has the full range of EAAs, and is second only to whey in terms of leucine content.

Compared to the other types of protein, egg protein is the easiest to digest. How-ever, it may not keep you as satiated as the other types of protein powders do, because the egg yolk has been removed.

Pea protein

Pea protein powder is a little newer on the playing field, but it already has excel-lent research behind it. Studies show that it provides the same protein nutrition as whey over three months.

Pea protein is an excellent option if you can't eat milk or eggs or you have a lot of allergies. It's easy to digest compared to the other plant-based proteins and is readily available to your muscles. However, like casein, pea protein is a slow-digesting type of protein, so it's not the best idea for a pre-workout source of energy.

WARNING

Pea protein is not a complete protein, meaning that although it does have all the BCAAs, it does not include all the EAAs. Therefore, even more so than milk-based proteins, pea protein should not be the primary source of protein in your diet.

Other plant-based proteins

There are a host of other plant-based proteins, including

>> Soy

>> Hemp

>> Brown rice

>> Mixed varieties, including chia, flax, and others

Although soy is a faster-acting protein, studies show it does not have as much of a muscle-building effect as either casein or whey proteins. Brown rice has generally been thought to be less effective than whey protein, although one study showed equivalent results after two months of weight training in active young men. There is even less research on the other plant-based proteins, suggesting that, as of now, pea protein should be the go-to if you choose a plant-based option.

TIP

Supplements are just that — supplements. Most of your protein should come from a well-rounded keto diet, and if you're eating adequate amounts of protein for your activity level, you may not need more. However, protein powders are a good option if you do resistance-type exercises and you're wanting to build more muscle mass while reducing fat.

Creatine

Creatine is one of the most well-studied supplements for muscle growth. This chemical is a crucial component of the energy cycle in cells, allowing muscles to recover quickly, which in turn permits you to push harder and longer during exercise. It has the following benefits:

>> **It stimulates ATP stores in your muscles so you can improve strength and speed in high-intensity (anaerobic) exercises like sprints and heavy weight lifting.** Studies show that there is an average of 5 percent increase in strength and power when supplementing with creatine.

>> **It increases muscle gains by swelling water mass in the muscle cells.**

>> **It increases the production of hormones like IGF-1 (insulin-like growth factor), which help increase MPS.** This hormone is essential for childhood growth and can increase muscle growth in adults.

>> **It decreases muscle breakdown over the long run.**

MCT oil

MCT oils are the one form of fat that may be useful around the time of a workout to help fuel your muscles. *Remember:* Fats are generally slow-absorbing, so they're unlikely to help feed your workout if you eat them right before. MCT oils are different from fat, however:

>> They're easily digested and fast absorbing because they're taken up by the liver quickly (similar to quick-absorbing carbs).

>> They're immediately converted to ketones so that your muscle can use them as an energy source.

>> They can help you become keto-adapted more quickly, making them an option for any keto athlete who wants to improve her muscles' fat-burning capabilities more quickly.

>> They may help reduce lactate buildup during anaerobic exercise, helping you to keep going longer on your workouts.

Also, MCT oils help you lose weight because they boost levels of the satiety hormone, leptin, preventing you from overeating. Studies show that it helps to rid you of pesky fat around the midsection, which is the worst type of fat for your health, and it helps boost gut-friendly bacteria, which are also crucial for maintaining a healthy weight. Finally, it's a great fuel for your brain so it can keep you focused on your goals during your intense workouts.

Generally, most people will use 1 or 2 tablespoons of MCT oil before a workout to help improve their energy.

TIP

You can always simply increase your intake of coconut oil because it's 65 percent MCT oil, depending on the purity and quality.

Ketones

Exogenous ketones are a fast way to get your ketone levels up to fuel your workouts. They contain beta-hydroxybutyrate (BHB) complex with a mineral. BHB is the most effective ketone and produces more energy than acetoacetate. It's also one of the primary sources of anti-inflammation in the keto diet. Generally, these supplements will either come in a powder form or a liquid.

The powder form is the ketone salts and is bound to a mineral. The complex minerals can be

>> Sodium

>> Calcium

>> Magnesium

>> Potassium

As such, these ketone salts may be an easy way to get extra minerals that you're depleted of, especially potassium or magnesium, where keto dieters are more likely to see deficiencies. The liquid form is a ketone ester. However, it's harder to buy these forms because they're generally used for research purposes.

Adding ketone salts may help boost your energy during your workout because it will add more ketones as a fuel to your active muscle. Ketone salts may specifically aid the cyclical keto dieter who finds it difficult to get back into ketosis after the carb days.

Generally, you should take 8 to 12 grams of ketone salts about an hour before your workout to experience their benefits. Some people choose to combine MCT oils with ketones for an extra boost.

Other supplements for overall health

These options aren't specific to working out. Many people take them regularly just for health or other benefits, but they can add a boost to your workouts. If you're on regular medication, always talk with your doctor before adding any supplements:

>> **A daily multivitamin:** This is crucial for most keto dieters because it can be easy to fail to get all the vitamins and minerals you need as you're transitioning into keto and even after. Make sure you take a multivitamin that includes all the common minerals that can be deficient in keto, like potassium, magnesium, and zinc.

MONEY DOWN THE DRAIN

Beta-hydroxy beta-methylbutyrate (HMB) is a metabolite of leucine, which is one of the BCAAs that is known for its benefits on MPS. Studies have shown that HMB is a useful supplement in untrained athletes or elderly people new to resistance training who are experiencing muscle loss. However, if your goal is significant muscle gain and you're a trained athlete or bodybuilder, HMB offers negligible benefits. A recent *meta-analysis* (a combination of multiple studies) of HMB showed no benefit in terms of performance gains (in bench press and leg press) or improvement in terms of fat loss or muscle gains.

>> **Caffeine:** Caffeine is found in many of the workout supplements out there, but if you already drink a morning cup of joe each day, you probably don't need to purchase additional caffeine supplements. However, if you don't like the taste of coffee or you don't consume it regularly, you may notice some benefits with about 150 to 200 milligrams of caffeine; this dose not only increases mental clarity, but also can help burn an extra 150 or more calories while you work out if weight loss is your goal.

>> **L-theanine:** L-theanine is a naturally occurring amino acid found in both black and green teas. Its claim to fame is its ability to improve relaxation without causing drowsiness. It has also been shown to improve mental focus, decrease anxiety, and improve working memory. Generally, 200 to 400 milligrams is an effective dose per day.

>> **Fish oil:** Omega-3 fish oil is a great source of anti-inflammatory nutrients. Generally, the recommendations are to get 1 to 3 grams of omega-3s per day for health, with a ratio of 2:1 eicosapentaenoic acid (EPA) to docosahexaenoic acid (DHA). Some studies show that in addition to its heart-healthy benefits, omega-3s may boost muscle building, as well as decrease the dreaded delayed-onset muscle soreness after an intense workout.

5

Keto Recipes

Chapter **14**

Breakfast: Starting Your Day the Keto Way

You've probably heard that breakfast is the most important meal of the day, and a number of scientific studies support this statement. The average person goes the longest time without eating in the period between supper and breakfast. What you eat when "breaking your fast" sets your day up for either success or failure: Eat a heavy load of carbs, and you'll end up lethargic, unproductive, and struggling with energy surges and drop-offs throughout the day.

Eggs are obviously the easiest and most natural choice for keto-friendly breakfasts, and we've included several recipes in this chapter that make these delicious offerings the central part of the recipe. However, you can only eat so many eggs before you start to realize you're not able to look a chicken in the eye anymore.

To help you avoid this burnout, we've assembled a variety of carb-replacement recipes that are so good, you may even forget you're on keto. These include pancakes, toast, waffles, and shakes — items you may have written off entirely and assumed you'd seen the last of on Earth.

We believe keto has the power to change your life, but that shouldn't require you to *give up* your life. Start off each day right with a low-carb recipe that tastes strikingly similar to the original recipe, is healthier, and will fuel you for much longer than other, high-carb breakfast options.

Blueberry Almond Pancakes

PREP TIME: 5 MIN	COOK TIME: 10 MIN	YIELD: 2 SERVINGS

INGREDIENTS

1 cup almond flour

1 teaspoon baking powder

Pinch salt

3 large eggs

2 tablespoons unsweetened almond milk

½ teaspoon vanilla extract

1 tablespoon avocado oil

½ cup frozen blueberries

2 tablespoons unsalted butter

DIRECTIONS

1 In a medium bowl, whisk together the almond flour, baking powder, and salt.

2 In a separate bowl, whisk together the eggs, almond milk, and vanilla extract.

3 Pour the wet ingredients into the dry ingredients while whisking, and stir until smooth.

4 Heat and lightly grease a griddle pan and spoon the batter onto the pan to make six 5-inch pancakes.

5 Sprinkle some blueberries into the wet batter of each pancake, dividing them evenly among the pancakes.

6 Cook the pancakes until bubbles form in the surface of the batter.

7 Carefully flip the pancakes and cook until golden brown underneath.

8 Slide the pancakes onto a plate and top with butter to serve.

PER SERVING: *Calories 614 (From Fat 484); Fat 54g (Saturated 12g); Cholesterol 310mg; Sodium 409mg; Carbohydrate 17g (Dietary Fiber 7g); Net Carbohydrate 10g; Protein 22g.*

Avocado Cloud Toast

PREP TIME: 10 MIN	COOK TIME: 30 MIN	YIELD: 2 SERVINGS

INGREDIENTS

2 large eggs, separated

¼ teaspoon garlic powder

Pinch cream of tartar

1 ounce cream cheese, cubed

½ cup mayonnaise

2 teaspoons fresh lemon juice

1 large avocado

4 slices fresh tomato

Salt, to taste

Fresh cracked pepper, to taste

DIRECTIONS

1 Preheat the oven to 300 degrees and line a baking sheet with parchment paper.

2 In a medium bowl, beat the egg whites and cream of tartar with a hand mixer on medium speed until stiff peaks form, about 30 seconds.

3 In a separate bowl, beat together the cream cheese, egg yolk and garlic powder until pale in color and well combined.

4 Gently fold the egg whites into the cream cheese mixture.

5 Spoon the mixture onto the baking sheet in 4-inch circles, spacing them 1 to 2 inches apart.

6 Bake for 20 to 30 minutes until lightly golden brown. Keep an eye on the buns as they bake. Then remove from the oven and cool completely.

7 In a small bowl, whisk together the mayonnaise and fresh lemon juice.

8 Open and pit the avocado; then cut it into quarters and slice thin.

9 Toast the buns and spread with the mayonnaise mixture.

10 Top each bun with 1 slice of tomato and 1 quarter of the sliced avocado.

11 Season with salt and pepper before serving.

PER SERVING: *Calories 665 (From Fat 592); Fat 66g (Saturated 13g); Cholesterol 225mg; Sodium 767mg; Carbohydrate 12g (Dietary Fiber 7g); Net Carbohydrate 5g; Protein 10g.*

Chocolate Chip Waffles

PREP TIME: 15 MIN | COOK TIME: 10 MIN | YIELD: 2 SERVINGS

INGREDIENTS

2 large eggs, separated

3 tablespoons low-carb vanilla protein powder

2 tablespoons unsalted butter, melted

1 tablespoon powdered erythritol

½ teaspoon vanilla extract

Pinch salt

2 tablespoons stevia-sweetened chocolate chips

Sugar-free maple syrup, to taste

DIRECTIONS

1 In a medium bowl, beat the egg whites until stiff peaks form.

2 In a separate bowl, whisk together the protein powder, butter, egg yolks, erythritol, vanilla extract, and salt.

3 Fold the egg whites into the protein powder mixture, and then fold in the chocolate chips.

4 Grease and preheat a waffle iron, and then cook the batter according to the manufacturer's instructions, until golden brown.

5 Remove the waffles to a plate and top with sugar-free maple syrup to serve.

PER SERVING: *Calories 244 (From Fat 171); Fat 19g (Saturated 10g); Cholesterol 221mg; Sodium 171mg; Carbohydrate 5g (Dietary Fiber 2g); Net Carbohydrate 3g; Protein 15g.*

Breakfast Taco with Cheesy Shells

PREP TIME: 10 MIN | **COOK TIME: 15 MIN** | **YIELD: 2 SERVINGS**

INGREDIENTS

1 cup shredded mozzarella cheese

½ cup shredded cheddar cheese

4 slices bacon

6 large eggs

2 tablespoons heavy cream

Salt, to taste

Pepper, to taste

½ medium avocado, diced

1 small tomato, chopped

DIRECTIONS

1 Place a wooden spoon over a bowl and set it aside.

2 Heat a large skillet over medium-high heat.

3 In a medium bowl, combine the mozzarella and cheddar cheeses.

4 Sprinkle ¼ cup of the cheese blend in a circle in the middle of the skillet.

5 Let the cheese melt and brown; then flip and cook until the underside is browned.

6 Use a spatula to remove the cheese from the skillet and drape it over the wooden spoon to cool into a taco shell shape; repeat for the rest of the cheese.

7 Cook the bacon in the same skillet until crisp; then drain on paper towel and chop.

8 Grease another skillet and heat it over medium-high heat.

9 In a small bowl, whisk together the eggs, cream, salt, and pepper.

10 Pour the eggs into the skillet and cook for 3 to 5 minutes, stirring occasionally to scramble.

11 Place the taco shells upright on two plates.

12 Spoon the eggs into the shells; top with avocado, tomato, and chopped bacon to serve.

PER SERVING: *Calories 706 (From Fat 487); Fat 54g (Saturated 24g); Cholesterol 670mg; Sodium 1,313mg; Carbohydrate 9g (Dietary Fiber 2g); Net Carbohydrate 7g; Protein 46g.*

Strawberries and Cream Shake

PREP TIME: 5 MIN	COOK TIME: NONE	YIELD: 1 SERVING

INGREDIENTS

½ cup fresh strawberries

½ cup unsweetened almond milk

½ cup heavy cream

½ teaspoon vanilla extract

3 to 4 ice cubes

Liquid stevia extract, to taste

2 tablespoons sugar-free or unsweetened whipped cream, optional

DIRECTIONS

1 Wash the strawberries and remove the stems; then chop them coarsely.

2 In a blender, combine the almond milk, heavy cream, and vanilla extract.

3 Add the strawberries and ice, and then blend until smooth.

4 Sweeten to taste with liquid stevia, and then blend until smooth once more.

5 Pour into a glass and top with whipped cream to serve, if desired.

PER SERVING: *Calories 467 (From Fat 415); Fat 46g (Saturated 28g); Cholesterol 164mg; Sodium 137mg; Carbohydrate 11g (Dietary Fiber 3g); Net Carbohydrate 8g; Protein 5g.*

Mini Baked Quiches

PREP TIME: 10 MIN	COOK TIME: 25 MIN	YIELD: 4 SERVINGS

INGREDIENTS

1 teaspoon olive oil

8 ounces white mushrooms, diced

4 ounces diced tomatoes

¼ cup diced red onion

2 cloves minced garlic

6 large eggs

½ cup heavy cream

1 tablespoon fresh chopped parsley

Salt, to taste

Pepper, to taste

1 cup shredded mozzarella cheese

DIRECTIONS

1 Preheat the oven to 350 degrees, and grease a muffin pan with cooking spray.

2 In a large skillet, heat the oil over medium heat.

3 Add the mushrooms, tomatoes, red onion, and garlic; then cook until tender, about 6 to 8 minutes.

4 In a medium bowl, whisk together the eggs, cream, parsley, salt, and pepper until pale.

5 Stir in the cooked vegetables and mozzarella cheese.

6 Spoon the batter into the prepared pan, filling the cups evenly.

7 Bake for 22 to 25 minutes until the eggs are set and the tops are lightly browned.

8 Cool completely; then remove from the tin and store in an airtight container in the refrigerator.

PER SERVING: *Calories 329 (From Fat 232); Fat 26g (Saturated 13g); Cholesterol 342mg; Sodium 445mg; Carbohydrate 7g (Dietary Fiber 1g); Net Carbohydrate 6g; Protein 18g.*

Goat Cheese Frittata

PREP TIME: 15 MIN	COOK TIME: 30 MIN	YIELD: 4 SERVINGS

INGREDIENTS

16 medium spears asparagus

2 tablespoons olive oil

4 ounces sliced white mushrooms

12 large eggs

½ cup heavy cream

2 cloves minced garlic

Salt, to taste

Pepper, to taste

4 ounces crumbled goat cheese

2 green onions, sliced thin

DIRECTIONS

1 Trim the ends from the asparagus and cut into 2-inch pieces.

2 In a 10-inch cast-iron skillet, heat the oil over medium-high heat.

3 Add the mushrooms and asparagus, and sauté for 3 to 4 minutes, until browned.

4 In a medium bowl, whisk together the eggs, cream, garlic, salt, and pepper.

5 Pour the liquid mixture into the skillet and sprinkle with goat cheese and green onion.

6 Bake for 30 minutes at 375 degrees, until set; then cut into wedges to serve.

PER SERVING: *Calories 505 (From Fat 366); Fat 41g (Saturated 18g); Cholesterol 622mg; Sodium 531mg; Carbohydrate 7g (Dietary Fiber 2g); Net Carbohydrate 5g; Protein 28g.*

Sweet Raspberry Porridge

PREP TIME: 5 MIN	COOK TIME: 8 MIN	YIELD: 2 SERVINGS

INGREDIENTS

2 cups unsweetened almond milk

¼ cup ground flaxseed

¼ cup coconut flour

⅔ cup fresh raspberries

1 teaspoon vanilla extract

8 to 10 drops liquid stevia extract, to taste

DIRECTIONS

1 In a small saucepan, warm the almond milk over medium heat.

2 When the almond milk starts steaming, whisk in the flaxseed and coconut flour until well combined.

3 Stir in the raspberries and cook until thickened, about 10 minutes.

4 Remove from heat and stir in the vanilla extract.

5 Sweeten with liquid stevia to taste and spoon into bowls to serve.

PER SERVING: *Calories 188 (From Fat 88); Fat 10g (Saturated 2g); Cholesterol 0mg; Sodium 211mg; Carbohydrate 19g (Dietary Fiber 13g); Net Carbohydrate 6g; Protein 7g.*

Chapter **15**

Keto Lunches

S taying on track with the keto diet requires rethinking the way you do lunch. It's actually not that difficult, but because cooking with fat requires a different set of skills than cooking with carbs does, you'll have to challenge some of your basic habits when it comes to meal prep. You can't default to sandwiches, and ordering in pizza isn't typically an option.

What you'll find, however, is that when you begin cooking intentionally with an eye toward health, not only will your nutrition take a noticeable turn for the better, but you'll start to experience a much higher premium on taste. Unfortunately, most people settle for a boring, bland, less-than-healthy lunch at work, almost as if it's something they have to endure rather than enjoy. That isn't the case with keto-friendly foods.

All the lunchtime recipes we include in this chapter have passed some rigorous tests: They have to keep you on your macros, be filled with healthy ingredients, be easy to prepare initially, and be just as simple to enjoy in a restricted work environment. One of the most important criteria of a successful keto meal is the taste, though. We love how much flavor fat adds to food, and we feel confident that, after just a little bit of adjustment, your taste buds will no longer crave the over-preserved carbs that used to fill your midday meal and you'll actually prefer the delicious, varied, rich flavor of fat-filled foods.

Chicken-Avocado Salad

PREP TIME: 10 MIN | COOK TIME: 12 MIN | YIELD: 1 SERVING

INGREDIENTS

One 3-ounce boneless chicken thigh

Salt and pepper, to taste

1 small celery stalk, diced

1 tablespoon diced red onion

½ teaspoon fresh chopped parsley

1 cup diced avocado

⅓ cup sour cream

1 teaspoon fresh lemon juice

Pinch garlic powder

DIRECTIONS

1 Grease and preheat a grill pan to medium-high heat.

2 Season the chicken with salt and pepper and then add to the grill pan.

3 Cook for 5 to 6 minutes on each side, until cooked through, then remove. Allow the chicken to cool a little and then shred it.

4 In a mixing bowl, combine the celery, red onion, and fresh parsley.

5 Toss in the diced avocado and shredded chicken.

6 Add the sour cream, lemon juice, and garlic powder, and toss well to combine.

7 Season with salt and pepper to taste and serve.

PER SERVING: *Calories 506 (From Fat 389); Fat 43g (Saturated 13g); Cholesterol 112mg; Sodium 417mg; Carbohydrate 17g (Dietary Fiber 11g); Net Carbohydrate 6g; Protein 18g.*

Cheeseburger Crepes

PREP TIME: 10 MIN | COOK TIME: 20 MIN | YIELD: 2 SERVINGS

INGREDIENTS

2 tablespoons olive oil

6 ounces 80 percent lean ground beef

½ small yellow onion, diced

1 ounce shredded cheddar cheese

1 tablespoon sugar-free ketchup

2 tablespoons mayonnaise
2 large eggs

2 ounces cream cheese, softened

DIRECTIONS

1 In a greased skillet over medium heat, cook the ground beef and onion for 5 minutes.

2 Stir in the cheddar cheese, ketchup, and mayonnaise; then spoon into a bowl and set aside.

3 In a medium bowl, make a batter by beating together the eggs and cream cheese until smooth and well combined.

4 Grease a large skillet and heat it over high heat.

5 Spoon about ½ of the batter into the skillet, tilting to coat it evenly, and cook for 2 minutes.

6 Carefully flip the crepe and fry for another 2 minutes, until lightly browned.

7 Remove the crepe to a plate and keep warm while you use the rest of the batter.

8 Spoon the cheeseburger mixture into the crepes and roll them up; then cut in half to serve.

PER SERVING: *Calories 600 (From Fat 474); Fat 53g (Saturated 17g); Cholesterol 291mg; Sodium 455mg; Carbohydrate 7g (Dietary Fiber 0g); Net Carbohydrate 7g; Protein 27g.*

Meatball Marinara Bake

PREP TIME: 15 MIN	COOK TIME: 30 MIN	YIELD: 8 SERVINGS

INGREDIENTS

1½ pounds 80 percent lean ground beef

4 large eggs

1 cup grated parmesan cheese

¼ cup diced yellow onion

2 tablespoons almond flour

2 cloves minced garlic

Salt and pepper, to taste

1 tablespoon olive oil

2 cups no-sugar-added marinara sauce

2 cups shredded mozzarella cheese

Fresh chopped parsley, to serve

DIRECTIONS

1 Preheat the oven to 350 degrees, and grease a 9-x-9-inch casserole dish with cooking spray.

2 In a large bowl, combine the beef, eggs, parmesan cheese, onion, almond flour, and garlic.

3 Season with salt and pepper; then combine and shape by hand into 16 small meatballs.

4 Grease a large skillet and heat over high heat; add the meatballs.

5 Sear the meatballs on all sides for 3 to 5 minutes, until browned.

6 Pour the marinara sauce into the casserole dish and add the meatballs.

7 Top with shredded mozzarella, and bake for 20 minutes.

8 Place the casserole under the broiler for 2 minutes to brown the cheese.

9 Garnish with parsley to serve.

PER SERVING: *Calories 356 (From Fat 211); Fat 23g (Saturated 10g); Cholesterol 176mg; Sodium 767mg; Carbohydrate 6g (Dietary Fiber 2g); Net Carbohydrate 4g; Protein 29g.*

Cashew Chicken Stir-Fry

PREP TIME: 10 MIN	COOK TIME: 20 MIN	YIELD: 4 SERVINGS

INGREDIENTS

Two 7-ounce bags Miracle Noodle Rice

Salt and pepper, to taste

1 teaspoon coconut oil

1 pound boneless chicken thighs, chopped

2 tablespoons canned coconut milk

2 tablespoons soy sauce

20 small spears asparagus, sliced

½ cup whole cashews

1 teaspoon chili garlic sauce, optional

2 cloves minced garlic

DIRECTIONS

1 Empty the Miracle Noodle Rice into a strainer and rinse well with cool water.

2 Grease a large skillet with cooking spray and heat over medium heat.

3 Add the Miracle Noodle Rice and season with salt and pepper. Sauté until heated through.

4 In a separate skillet, heat the coconut oil over medium heat.

5 Add the chicken to the coconut oil and cook until browned, stirring often, about 4 to 5 minutes.

6 Pour the coconut milk and soy sauce into the skillet with the chicken.

7 Add the asparagus, cashews, chili garlic sauce, and garlic and simmer for 6 to 8 minutes, stirring occasionally.

8 Stir in the Miracle Noodle Rice and simmer for 2 minutes until heated through.

PER SERVING: *Calories 313 (From Fat 183); Fat 20g (Saturated 7g); Cholesterol 106mg; Sodium 657mg; Carbohydrate 11g (Dietary Fiber 5g); Net Carbohydrate 6g; Protein 22g.*

Creamy Shrimp and Vegetable Curry

PREP TIME: 5 MIN	COOK TIME: 10 MIN	YIELD: 2 SERVINGS

INGREDIENTS

1 tablespoon coconut oil

1 medium zucchini, diced

1 cup sliced mushrooms

½ small yellow onion, chopped

1 clove minced garlic

12 ounces large shrimp, peeled and deveined

2 tablespoons shelled edamame

4 ounces cream cheese, softened

1 tablespoon soy sauce

1 teaspoon red curry paste

½ teaspoon turmeric

½ cup chicken broth

¼ cup fresh chopped cilantro

DIRECTIONS

1 In a large skillet, heat the oil over medium heat.

2 Add the zucchini, mushrooms, onion, and garlic; then stir-fry until tender, about 6 to 7 minutes.

3 Place the shrimp in the skillet in a single layer, and cook 1 to 2 minutes on each side, until pink.

4 Stir in the edamame, cream cheese, soy sauce, curry paste, turmeric, and broth.

5 Cook for 2 minutes or until the cream cheese is melted; adjust the seasoning to taste.

6 Spoon into bowls and serve with fresh cilantro.

PER SERVING: *Calories 425 (From Fat 252); Fat 28g (Saturated 17g); Cholesterol 265mg; Sodium 1,031mg; Carbohydrate 12g (Dietary Fiber 3g); Net Carbohydrate 9g; Protein 34g.*

Loaded Cobb Salad

PREP TIME: 10 MIN	COOK TIME: 5 MIN	YIELD: 2 SERVINGS

INGREDIENTS

4 slices bacon

2 cups fresh baby spinach

2 large eggs, hardboiled and chopped

1 small avocado, pitted and sliced

Salt and pepper, to taste

1 tablespoon heavy cream

1 tablespoon mayonnaise

1 tablespoon sour cream

½ teaspoon fresh chopped chives

½ teaspoon fresh chopped parsley

¼ teaspoon fresh lemon juice

Pinch garlic powder

Pinch onion powder

DIRECTIONS

1 In a large skillet over medium heat, cook the bacon until crisp.

2 Drain on paper towels and chop coarsely; set aside.

3 Divide the spinach between two salad plates or bowls.

4 Top each salad with half of the eggs, avocado, and bacon; season with salt and pepper.

5 In a small bowl, whisk together the remaining ingredients, and then drizzle over the salads to serve.

PER SERVING: *Calories 355 (From Fat 269); Fat 30g (Saturated 8g); Cholesterol 220mg; Sodium 722mg; Carbohydrate 9g (Dietary Fiber 5g); Net Carbohydrate 4g; Protein 14g.*

Lemon Kale Salad

PREP TIME: 10 MIN	COOK TIME: NONE	YIELD: 2 SERVINGS

INGREDIENTS

4 ounces fresh kale

¼ cup olive oil

3 tablespoons fresh lemon juice

1 tablespoon fresh lemon zest

2 cloves minced garlic

Salt and pepper, to taste

¼ cup slivered almonds

2 ounces feta cheese, crumbled

DIRECTIONS

1 Rinse the kale in fresh water; pat dry.

2 Trim away the thick stems and tear the leaves into bite-size pieces.

3 Place the kale in a salad bowl with the olive oil, lemon juice, lemon zest, garlic, salt, and pepper.

4 Toss to coat; then massage the kale for a few minutes to soften.

5 Add the almonds and feta cheese, and toss to combine.

PER SERVING: Calories 431 (From Fat 359); Fat 40g (Saturated 9g); Cholesterol 25mg; Sodium 630mg; Carbohydrate 13g (Dietary Fiber 3g); Net Carbohydrate 9g; Protein 10g.

Chicken Pizza Casserole

PREP TIME: 15 MIN	COOK TIME: 30 MIN	YIELD: 4 SERVINGS

INGREDIENTS

1 pound boneless chicken thighs

1 tablespoon olive oil

2 large zucchini, cubed

12 ounces whole-milk ricotta cheese

4 ounces sliced pepperoni, divided

2 cloves minced garlic

Salt and pepper, to taste

1 cup shredded mozzarella cheese

¼ cup grated parmesan

DIRECTIONS

1 Preheat the oven to 350 degrees and grease a 9-x-13-inch glass baking dish.

2 Cook the chicken thighs in an oiled skillet over medium heat until cooked through.

3 Remove the chicken to a cutting board and shred with two forks.

4 In a large bowl, toss together the shredded chicken with the zucchini, the ricotta cheese, half the pepperoni, the garlic, the salt, and the pepper.

5 Spread the mixture in the baking dish and bake for 20 minutes.

6 Sprinkle with mozzarella and parmesan, and then top with the remaining pepperoni.

7 Bake for another 5 to 10 minutes, until the cheese is melted.

PER SERVING: Calories 631 (From Fat 418); Fat 47g (Saturated 20g); Cholesterol 205mg; Sodium 1,052mg; Carbohydrate 9g (Dietary Fiber 2g); Net Carbohydrate 7g; Protein 44g.

Chapter **16**

Keto Dinners

B reakfast and lunch are often eaten in a rush, but dinner is where you get to let your culinary passion and skill shine, and we urge you to embrace it! You're already changing the ingredients you use and exploring different recipes and ways of cooking, so go all the way! Pull out that blender, food processor, or mixer and really explore all the ways you can exploit the full range of your taste buds.

In the first few weeks of being on keto, virtually everything you cook will be new if you've never gone low carb before. Pick your favorites, put aside the ones you prefer less, and keep exploring. We understand that it can be exhausting to try a new recipe every single night, so when you have a solid base of recipes you're comfortable with, a great way to consistently and sustainably broaden your horizons is to pick one night a week where you'll try something new. Go all the way with it: Limiting your exploration to one or two nights a week allows you to really look forward to it, anticipating the ingredients you'll need and the side dishes you'll make. We've had times where we planned a new meal over the course of three or four days, and then spent several hours in the kitchen making sure it was just right while enjoying each other's company.

Keto allows you to explore a broad range of culinary abilities, tools, preparation methods, and a much more expansive list of ingredients than you might have used before. You'll find that the extensive number of ways you can use butter, for example, may completely change your mind-set with regards to what's within the realm of the possible in a frying pan.

Parmesan Meatballs with Zoodles

PREP TIME: 10 MIN	COOK TIME: 15 MIN	YIELD: 2 SERVINGS

INGREDIENTS

½ pound 80 percent lean ground beef

¼ cup plus 2 tablespoons grated parmesan cheese

2 tablespoons almond flour

1 clove minced garlic

1 large egg

Salt and pepper, to taste

½ cup sugar-free pasta sauce

1 tablespoon fresh chopped basil

1 medium zucchini, spiralized

1 tablespoon fresh chopped parsley

DIRECTIONS

1 In a large bowl, combine the beef, ¼ cup of parmesan cheese, almond flour, garlic, and egg.

2 Season with salt and pepper and then mix well by hand and shape into 1-inch balls.

3 Grease a large skillet with cooking spray and heat over high heat.

4 Add the meatballs and sear on all sides; reduce the heat and add the pasta sauce and basil.

5 Simmer, covered, for 10 minutes while you spiralize the zucchini noodles.

6 Cook the noodles in a greased pan over medium heat for 2 minutes until cooked through.

7 Serve the meatballs over a bed of zucchini noodles and spoon the extra sauce over them.

8 Garnish with the remaining 2 tablespoons of fresh grated parmesan cheese and parsley to serve.

PER SERVING: *Calories 381 (From Fat 212); Fat 24g (Saturated 9g); Cholesterol 177mg; Sodium 928mg; Carbohydrate 10g (Dietary Fiber 4g); Net Carbohydrate 6g; Protein 32g.*

Salmon with Avocado Lime Puree

| PREP TIME: 10 MIN | COOK TIME: 20 MIN | YIELD: 2 SERVINGS |

INGREDIENTS

1 cup cauliflower, chopped

2 tablespoons fresh chopped cilantro

1 clove minced garlic

Salt and pepper, to taste

1 medium avocado

2 tablespoons canned coconut milk

1 tablespoon fresh lime juice

1 teaspoon coconut oil

Two 6-ounce boneless salmon fillets

2 tablespoons diced red onion

DIRECTIONS

1 Place the cauliflower in a food processor and pulse into rice-like grains.

2 Grease a large skillet and heat it over low heat; then add the cauliflower, cilantro, and garlic.

3 Season with salt and pepper and cook, covered, for 8 minutes, until tender.

4 In a blender, combine the avocado, coconut milk, and lime juice and season with salt and pepper.

5 Blend until smooth and creamy; then set aside.

6 In a large skillet, heat the coconut oil over medium heat.

7 Season the salmon with salt and pepper.

8 Add the salmon to the skillet and cook for 4 to 5 minutes on each side, until just cooked through.

9 Spoon the cauliflower onto plates, top with a salmon fillet, and garnish with avocado lime puree and diced red onion.

PER SERVING: *Calories 411 (From Fat 211); Fat 24g (Saturated 7g); Cholesterol 80mg; Sodium 442mg; Carbohydrate 13g (Dietary Fiber 4g); Net Carbohydrate 9g; Protein 40g.*

Pan-Seared Pork Chops with Apple

PREP TIME: 10 MIN	COOK TIME: 20 MIN	YIELD: 2 SERVINGS

INGREDIENTS

Two 6-ounce boneless pork loin chops

½ teaspoon dried thyme

Salt and pepper, to taste

½ cup sliced apple

2 sprigs fresh rosemary

1 tablespoon olive oil

2 cups cauliflower, chopped

¼ cup grated parmesan cheese

2 tablespoons unsalted butter

2 tablespoons heavy cream

DIRECTIONS

1 Season the pork chops with thyme, salt, and pepper.

2 In a large skillet, heat the oil over high heat and add the pork; sear on both sides.

3 Lower the flame and then top the pork with the apples and rosemary.

4 Cover and cook for 6 to 8 minutes until just cooked through.

5 In the meantime, place a steamer insert in a medium saucepan with 1 inch of water; add the cauliflower.

6 Bring the water to a boil and steam the cauliflower for 8 minutes until tender.

7 Drain the cauliflower and then mash it with the parmesan cheese, butter, and heavy cream in a bowl; season with salt and pepper to taste.

8 Spoon the mashed cauliflower onto plates and serve with the pork chops.

PER SERVING: *Calories 582 (From Fat 386); Fat 43g (Saturated 19g); Cholesterol 155mg; Sodium 579mg; Carbohydrate 9g (Dietary Fiber 3g); Net Carbohydrate 6g; Protein 39g.*

Extra-Crispy Chicken Thighs

PREP TIME: 10 MIN | COOK TIME: 25 MIN | YIELD: 2 SERVINGS

INGREDIENTS

4 boneless chicken thighs, skin on

1 tablespoon fresh lemon juice

½ teaspoon garlic powder

Salt and pepper, to taste

1 medium zucchini

1 teaspoon olive oil

2 cloves minced garlic

4 tablespoons unsalted butter

DIRECTIONS

1 Preheat the oven to 350 degrees and place a cooling rack over a rimmed baking sheet.

2 Brush the chicken thighs with lemon juice, and then sprinkle with garlic powder, salt, and pepper.

3 Place the chicken thighs on the rack and bake for 20 minutes.

4 In a large skillet over medium-high heat, sauté the zucchini in the olive oil until just tender.

5 Add the garlic and sauté for 30 seconds more; then season with salt and pepper.

6 Place 1 tablespoon of butter on each chicken thigh, and then broil until crispy.

7 Serve the chicken with the sautéed zucchini.

PER SERVING: *Calories 867 (From Fat 586); Fat 66g (Saturated 28g); Cholesterol 426mg; Sodium 537mg; Carbohydrate 6g (Dietary Fiber 1g); Net Carbohydrate 5g; Protein 63g.*

Marinara Poached Cod

PREP TIME: 5 MIN | **COOK TIME: 15 MIN** | **YIELD: 2 SERVINGS**

INGREDIENTS

2 tablespoons olive oil

½ cup sugar-free marinara sauce

1 tablespoon fresh chopped basil

2 cloves minced garlic

3 small bay leaves

Salt and pepper, to taste

Two 8-ounce cod fillets

1 teaspoon coconut oil

2 cups green beans, sliced

DIRECTIONS

1 In a saucepan, heat the olive oil, marinara sauce, basil, and garlic over medium heat.

2 Add the bay leaves, salt, and pepper, and simmer for 5 minutes.

3 Reduce the heat to low, and add the cod fillets.

4 Cover and cook for 10 minutes, flipping the fish once halfway through.

5 In a separate pan, sauté the green beans in coconut oil until tender.

6 When the cod is cooked through, serve with the green beans.

PER SERVING: *Calories 403 (From Fat 193); Fat 22g (Saturated 8g); Cholesterol 86mg; Sodium 705mg; Carbohydrate 13g (Dietary Fiber 5g); Net Carbohydrate 8g; Protein 39g.*

Soy Glazed Chicken

PREP TIME: 35 MIN | COOK TIME: 20 MIN | YIELD: 2 SERVINGS

INGREDIENTS

¼ cup soy sauce

2 tablespoons fresh lemon juice

1 teaspoon fresh grated ginger

2 cloves minced garlic

1 jalapeño pepper, seeded and minced

4 boneless chicken thighs, skin on

2 tablespoons olive oil

2 cups green beans, sliced

DIRECTIONS

1 In a large bowl, whisk together the soy sauce, lemon juice, ginger, garlic, and jalapeño.

2 Toss in the chicken thighs and marinate for 30 minutes.

3 Heat the oil in a large skillet over medium heat.

4 Add the chicken thighs and cook for 8 to 10 minutes on each side.

5 Cook the green beans in another pan over medium-high heat until browned.

6 Serve the chicken with the green beans.

PER SERVING: *Calories 782 (From Fat 483); Fat 54g (Saturated 13g); Cholesterol 365mg; Sodium 673mg; Carbohydrate 9g (Dietary Fiber 4g); Net Carbohydrate 5g; Protein 64g.*

Chapter **17**

Sides

The focus of this chapter is on side dishes: delicious additions to your main dish that accentuate and complement the flavors you've already included on the table.

Side dishes are one of the most easily neglected aspects of any dietary change. People tend to focus on the main dish, simply because that's the centerpiece of the meal and where they're likely getting the majority of their calories. But sides really add that zest and full-bodied flavor to meals! Your palate is expanded, and the various tastes that sides bring to the table can make or break a new dish.

Some of the recipes in this chapter take old favorites (like mashed potatoes) and introduce ways to prepare them in a keto-friendly fashion by using other ingredients, such as cauliflower. Don't dismiss these outright — substitute ingredients almost always taste different than the original dish, but this isn't always bad. One of our more popular dishes has become known as "crack slaw" because this variation of coleslaw is so delicious that it's downright addictive!

Side dishes are an excellent option to bring to parties or events where keto-friendly food may be in short supply. Sometimes we've even turned it into a game, seeing how many compliments we can get on a recipe before revealing that it's keto!

Oven-Roasted Brussels Sprouts and Parmesan

PREP TIME: 5 MIN	COOK TIME: 20 MIN	YIELD: 6 SERVINGS

INGREDIENTS

1¼ pounds fresh Brussels sprouts

¼ cup olive oil

1 teaspoon dried thyme

Salt and pepper, to taste

2 to 3 ounces parmesan cheese

DIRECTIONS

1 Preheat the oven to 450 degrees.

2 Trim the stems from the Brussels sprouts and cut them in half.

3 Place the Brussels sprouts in a large bowl, and toss with the olive oil, thyme, salt, and pepper.

4 Spread the Brussels sprouts on a baking sheet and roast for 15 to 20 minutes, until just browned.

5 Shave the parmesan cheese over the Brussels sprouts to serve.

PER SERVING: *Calories 158 (From Fat 109); Fat 12g (Saturated 3g); Cholesterol 8mg; Sodium 263mg; Carbohydrate 8g (Dietary Fiber 3g); Net Carbohydrate 5g; Protein 6g.*

Creamy Coleslaw

| PREP TIME: 10 MIN | COOK TIME: 5 MIN | YIELD: 4 SERVINGS |

INGREDIENTS

4 slices bacon

1 cup shredded green cabbage

1 cup shredded red cabbage

1 medium carrot, grated

½ cup mayonnaise

1 tablespoon heavy cream

1 teaspoon Dijon mustard

½ teaspoon garlic salt

Pepper, to taste

DIRECTIONS

1 In a medium skillet, cook the bacon over medium-high heat until crisp.

2 Remove the bacon to paper towel to drain; then chop the bacon coarsely.

3 Combine the rest of the ingredients in a bowl and mix well.

4 Chill until ready to serve; then top with the chopped bacon to garnish.

PER SERVING: *Calories 262 (From Fat 229); Fat 25g (Saturated 5g); Cholesterol 26mg; Sodium 483mg; Carbohydrate 5g (Dietary Fiber 1g); Net Carbohydrate 4g; Protein 4g.*

Cauliflower Mash and Browned Butter

PREP TIME: 5 MIN	COOK TIME: 20 MIN	YIELD: 6 SERVINGS

INGREDIENTS

1½ pounds cauliflower, chopped

¾ cups heavy cream

Salt and pepper, to taste

1 cup shredded cheddar cheese

3 ounces unsalted butter

DIRECTIONS

1 Place the cauliflower in a food processor and pulse into rice-like grains.

2 Pour the cauliflower rice into a large saucepan; then add the heavy cream.

3 Bring to a boil over medium heat; reduce the heat and simmer for 12 to 15 minutes, until the cauliflower is tender.

4 Season with salt and pepper, and then stir in the cheddar cheese. Set aside.

5 In a medium skillet, melt the butter over medium heat.

6 Cook the butter until it reaches a nice amber color; then drizzle over the cauliflower mash.

PER SERVING: *Calories 307 (From Fat 262); Fat 29g (Saturated 18g); Cholesterol 91mg; Sodium 243mg; Carbohydrate 6g (Dietary Fiber 2g); Net Carbohydrate 4g; Protein 8g.*

Curry Stir-Fried Cabbage

PREP TIME: 5 MIN	COOK TIME: 10 MIN	YIELD: 4 SERVINGS

INGREDIENTS

¼ cup unsalted butter

½ small yellow onion, diced

1½ pounds green cabbage, shredded

1 tablespoon white wine vinegar

1 tablespoon red curry paste

2 tablespoons water

3 cloves minced garlic

Salt and pepper

½ cup fresh chopped cilantro

DIRECTIONS

1 In a large skillet, heat the butter over medium-high heat.

2 Add the onions and sauté for 2 to 3 minutes, until just browned.

3 Stir in the cabbage and stir-fry for 5 to 6 minutes, until just softened.

4 Stir in the vinegar, curry paste, water, garlic, salt, and pepper, and sauté for 1 to 2 minutes.

5 Adjust the seasoning to taste, and top with fresh cilantro to serve.

PER SERVING: *Calories 172 (From Fat 112); Fat 13g (Saturated 7g); Cholesterol 31mg; Sodium 245mg; Carbohydrate 12g (Dietary Fiber 6g); Net Carbohydrate 6g; Protein 3g.*

Green Beans and Lemon Cream Sauce

PREP TIME: 5 MIN	COOK TIME: 5 MIN	YIELD: 4 SERVINGS

INGREDIENTS

¼ cup unsalted butter

10 ounces fresh green beans, trimmed

Salt and pepper, to taste

¼ cup heavy cream

1 tablespoon fresh lemon zest

¼ cup fresh chopped parsley

DIRECTIONS

1 In a large skillet, heat the butter over medium-high heat.

2 Add the green beans and sauté for 3 to 4 minutes, until tender-crisp. Season with salt and pepper to taste.

3 Spread the beans evenly in the skillet and pour in the heavy cream.

4 Simmer for 1 to 2 minutes, until thickened; then sprinkle with lemon zest and stir.

5 Adjust the seasoning to taste, and garnish with parsley to serve.

PER SERVING: *Calories 180 (From Fat 154); Fat 17g (Saturated 11g); Cholesterol 51mg; Sodium 156mg; Carbohydrate 7g (Dietary Fiber 3g); Net Carbohydrate 4g; Protein 2g.*

Buttery Garlic Mushrooms

PREP TIME: 15 MIN | COOK TIME: 15 MIN | YIELD: 4 SERVINGS

INGREDIENTS

¼ cup unsalted butter, melted

1 tablespoon fresh chopped thyme

1 teaspoon balsamic vinegar

2 cloves minced garlic

Salt and pepper, to taste

1½ pounds cremini mushrooms

Fresh chopped parsley

DIRECTIONS

1 Preheat the oven to 375 degrees, and line a rimmed baking sheet with foil.

2 In a medium bowl, whisk together the butter, thyme, vinegar, garlic, salt, and pepper.

3 Toss in the mushrooms until evenly coated.

4 Spread the mushrooms on the baking sheet and roast for 15 to 20 minutes until tender. Stir halfway through to help the mushrooms cook more evenly.

5 Garnish with parsley to serve.

PER SERVING: *Calories 143 (From Fat 104); Fat 12g (Saturated 7g); Cholesterol 31mg; Sodium 158mg; Carbohydrate 8g (Dietary Fiber 1g); Net Carbohydrate 7g; Protein 4g.*

Cheesy Baked Asparagus

PREP TIME: 10 MIN	COOK TIME: 30 MIN	YIELD: 4 SERVINGS

INGREDIENTS

1½ pounds medium asparagus spears

½ cup heavy cream

Salt and pepper, to taste

1 cup shredded mozzarella cheese

½ cup grated parmesan cheese

DIRECTIONS

1 Preheat the oven to 400 degrees, and grease a 9-x-13-inch glass baking dish.

2 Trim the ends from the asparagus and place the asparagus in the baking dish. Pour in the cream.

3 Season with salt and pepper, and then top with mozzarella and parmesan.

4 Bake for 25 minutes until the cheese is melted.

5 Place the dish under the broiler for 5 minutes to brown the cheese.

PER SERVING: *Calories 249 (From Fat 183); Fat 20g (Saturated 12g); Cholesterol 72mg; Sodium 487mg; Carbohydrate 5g (Dietary Fiber 2g); Net Carbohydrate 3g; Protein 13g.*

Chapter **18**

Appetizers and Snacks

Appetizers are some of the most amazing things in the world, especially if you're a foodie like we are. Think about it: They're literally recipes that are designed to be so delicious that their entire purpose is to make you want to eat more food! Appetizers are served at the beginning of the meal when your hunger is highest, your stomach is emptiest, and you're just ready to get going on a meal you've waited so long for. This requires the highest levels of satisfaction, and we're happy to report that keto appetizers deliver — and they deliver well.

Many traditional dishes in this category rely on small amounts of carbs: They're not really crucial to the food, but we've come to think of them as such. For example, when was the last time you were at a party and someone was eating guacamole, and then just stopped, looked around, and exclaimed in a loud voice: "Oh my gosh, these chips are amazing!" If you're hearing a compliment about chips and guacamole, it almost always centers on how delicious the dip itself is — the chip is just a delivery system for an explosion of flavor. You'll find that many appetizers are like this: If you want chicken wings, the focus is on the wings and the taste, which can be produced using either low-carb or high-carb methods and ingredients.

The dishes we present in this chapter focus on eliminating carbs from the mix while losing none of the flavor; in fact, we do our best to increase the "deliciousness factor" to the greatest extent possible. If the food we make is boring, that's a failure on our part, not a reflection of the ingredients available to us. Low-carb appetizers are another one of our favorite things to use to introduce non-keto-ers to the lifestyle, and we take a lot of pleasure in seeing people who thought keto was low-carb death-on-a-stick pull a complete 180 and ask for our recipe.

Using smaller dishes like these as snacks is another critical aspect of the keto approach. It can be challenging to get all your calories in if you're relying exclusively on full meals — fat is so filling that you'll find your portions decrease and you eat less as a result (remember that each gram of fat contains more than twice the energy of a gram of carbs). Eating less while you're on a diet focused around weight loss doesn't seem like it would be a problem, but remember that you *can* eat too little. The goal of weight loss is to eat enough to keep your metabolism high, but not so much that your body isn't digging into its fat stores and burning off that excess weight.

TIP

Snacks offer a great way to make minor adjustments to your macros and caloric intake as you're planning out your meals. When you create your meal list for the week and check it against your macros and find yourself a few hundred calories short, don't add another meal (which can bump your calories up to the point where you're no longer losing weight). Instead, just add a snack.

If you're doing intermittent fasting along with keto, concentrating your eating window to four to eight hours in a day can add an extra layer of difficulty when it comes to making sure you're eating enough. It's not impossible, by any means, but it does require some adjustment. A perfect way to satisfy this need is to add in some delicious snacks that cater to your cravings. The ones we offer in this chapter will give you an idea of what's possible, but there are scores of additional, full recipes on our website, www.tasteaholics.com/recipes/quick-bites, so be sure to follow up there when you're looking for other options.

Cheese Chips and Guacamole

PREP TIME: 5 MIN	COOK TIME: 12 MIN	YIELD: 2 SERVINGS

INGREDIENTS

½ cup shredded cheddar cheese

¼ teaspoon garlic powder

Pinch cayenne

1 medium avocado, chopped

½ small tomato, diced

1 tablespoon minced white onion

1 tablespoon fresh lime juice

1 tablespoon fresh chopped cilantro

¼ teaspoon ground cumin

Salt and pepper, to taste

DIRECTIONS

1 Preheat the oven to 425 degrees and line a baking sheet with parchment.

2 Sprinkle the shredded cheese in circles on the baking sheet, using about 1 tablespoon per circle, spacing them 1 inch apart.

3 Top the cheese with a pinch of garlic powder and cayenne.

4 Bake for 6 to 10 minutes, checking often, until the cheese is melted and bubbling.

5 Remove from the baking sheet and let cool until crisp.

6 In a bowl, mash the avocado and then stir in the tomato, onion, lime juice, cilantro, and cumin.

7 Season with salt and pepper.

8 Serve the guacamole with the cheddar cheese chips for dipping.

PER SERVING: *Calories 250 (From Fat 187); Fat 21g (Saturated 7g); Cholesterol 30mg; Sodium 469mg; Carbohydrate 10g (Dietary Fiber 3g); Net Carbohydrate 7g; Protein 10g.*

Pesto Bread Strips

PREP TIME: 10 MIN	COOK TIME: 20 MIN	YIELD: 8 SERVINGS

INGREDIENTS

½ cup almond flour

¼ cup coconut flour

1 teaspoon baking powder

½ teaspoon garlic powder

½ teaspoon salt

1½ cups shredded mozzarella cheese

5 tablespoons unsalted butter, softened

2 ounces pesto sauce

1 large egg, whisked well

DIRECTIONS

1 Preheat the oven to 350 degrees and line a baking sheet with parchment.

2 In a medium bowl, combine the almond flour, coconut flour, baking powder, garlic powder, and salt.

3 In a small saucepan, melt the cheese and butter on low heat and stir smooth.

4 Remove the cheese and butter from the heat and stir the mixture into the dry ingredients until it comes together in a dough.

5 Roll out the dough between two sheets of parchment to ¼-inch thickness.

6 Spread the pesto on top of the dough; then cut into 1-inch strips.

7 Place the bread strips on the baking sheet and brush with the egg.

8 Bake for 15 to 20 minutes, until golden brown; then serve warm.

PER SERVING: *Calories 226 (From Fat 176); Fat 20g (Saturated 9g); Cholesterol 61mg; Sodium 486mg; Carbohydrate 5g (Dietary Fiber 2g); Net Carbohydrate 3g; Protein 8g.*

Zucchini Chips with Ranch Dip

| PREP TIME: 10 MIN | COOK TIME: 2 HR | YIELD: 8 SERVINGS |

INGREDIENTS

1 cup mayonnaise

½ cup sour cream

1 tablespoon dried parsley

½ tablespoon dried chives

½ tablespoon dried dill

½ teaspoon garlic powder

Salt and pepper, to taste

4 cups sliced zucchini (very thin)

1 teaspoon dried oregano

1 tablespoon olive oil

Salt, to taste

DIRECTIONS

1 In a bowl, combine the mayonnaise, sour cream, parsley, chives, dill, and garlic powder.

2 Whisk well and season with salt and pepper; then chill until ready to use.

3 Preheat the oven to 225 degrees and line a baking sheet with parchment and grease with cooking spray.

4 In a medium bowl, toss the sliced zucchini with the oregano and olive oil; then spread on the baking sheet.

5 Sprinkle with salt; then bake for 1 to 2 hours until dried and crisp. Serve with the ranch dip.

PER SERVING: *Calories 239 (From Fat 224); Fat 25g (Saturated 5g); Cholesterol 18mg; Sodium 338mg; Carbohydrate 3g (Dietary Fiber 1g); Net Carbohydrate 2g; Protein 1g.*

Mini Caprese Skewers

| PREP TIME: 10 MIN | COOK TIME: NONE | YIELD: 4 SERVINGS |

INGREDIENTS

16 cherry tomatoes

4 ounces fresh mozzarella

8 large basil leaves, torn in half

2 tablespoons olive oil

2 tablespoons balsamic vinegar

Salt and pepper, to taste

DIRECTIONS

1 Cut the cherry tomatoes in half and cut the mozzarella into cubes.

2 Using wooden toothpicks create skewers with two tomato halves, two cubes of mozzarella, and one basil leaf torn in half.

3 Arrange the skewers on a plate or platter.

4 Drizzle with olive oil and balsamic vinegar; then season with salt and pepper to serve.

PER SERVING: *Calories 159 (From Fat 120); Fat 14g (Saturated 5g); Cholesterol 23mg; Sodium 172mg; Carbohydrate 4g (Dietary Fiber 1g); Net Carbohydrate 3g; Protein 5g.*

Crispy Baked Onion Rings

PREP TIME: 5 MIN	COOK TIME: 20 MIN	YIELD: 4 SERVINGS

INGREDIENTS

1 large yellow onion

1 cup almond flour

½ cup grated parmesan cheese

1 teaspoon garlic powder

1 teaspoon paprika

¼ teaspoon salt

1 large egg, whisked well

DIRECTIONS

1 Preheat the oven to 400 degrees and line a baking sheet with parchment.

2 Slice the onion into rings about ¼-inch thick.

3 In a bowl, combine the almond flour, parmesan cheese, garlic powder, paprika, and salt.

4 In a shallow dish, whisk the egg and then dip the onion rings into it.

5 Dredge the onion rings in the almond flour mixture; then place on the baking sheet.

6 Spray with cooking spray and bake for 15 to 20 minutes, until crisp and browned. Flip them halfway through, if needed.

PER SERVING: *Calories 240 (From Fat 164); Fat 18g (Saturated 3g); Cholesterol 55mg; Sodium 328mg; Carbohydrate 11g (Dietary Fiber 3g); Net Carbohydrate 8g; Protein 12g.*

Chapter 19

One-Pot Wonders

We lead busy lives. If we're not actively engaged in one activity, we're hurrying to the next or preparing for the one after that. The thought of putting everything aside and dedicating several hours to creating a delicious three-course meal is nice, but who has time for that?

Making food in a single pot, pan, or even baking sheet has numerous advantages — first and foremost, simplicity. Everything you need for your meal has been included in one dish, and these meals are known for being warm, hearty, and filling. You won't worry about walking away hungry from these meals. In fact, you may consider this chapter your "go-to" for those cold winter days where you just want the comfort of food that feels like home.

In addition to their uncomplicated nature, the level of convenience you find here is unparalleled. There's a reason we named this chapter "One-Pot Wonders": You can prepare a full meal with a variety of ingredients and tastes that fully fit your macros in a single dish. Few things have done more for making keto convenient than recipes that allow an entire meal to be prepared in a single container.

Steak Tenderloin with Crispy Kale

PREP TIME: 5 MIN	COOK TIME: 10 MIN	YIELD: 4 SERVINGS

INGREDIENTS

1 large bunch kale, thick stems removed and leaves torn into bite-size pieces

2 tablespoons olive oil

Salt and pepper, to taste

Four 8-ounce boneless beef tenderloin steaks

DIRECTIONS

1 In a large bowl, toss the kale with the olive oil; season with salt and pepper.

2 Line a rimmed baking sheet with parchment, and spread the kale on it.

3 Season the steaks with salt and pepper and place them on the baking sheet.

4 Broil on low for 2 to 3 minutes; then turn the steaks, stir the kale, and broil another 2 to 3 minutes.

5 Remove the baking sheet from the oven, and let the steaks rest 5 minutes before serving.

6 Serve the steaks hot with the crispy kale.

PER SERVING: *Calories 562 (From Fat 344); Fat 38g (Saturated 13g); Cholesterol 173mg; Sodium 256mg; Carbohydrate 5g (Dietary Fiber 1g); Net Carbohydrate 4g; Protein 48g.*

Butternut Squash Soup

PREP TIME: 5 MIN	COOK TIME: 45 MIN	YIELD: 4 SERVINGS

INGREDIENTS

1 pound, peeled and cubed butternut squash

1 tablespoon olive oil

Salt and pepper, to taste

2 cups chicken broth

½ cup canned coconut milk

1 tablespoon minced garlic

1 tablespoon fresh chopped thyme

¼ teaspoon ground cinnamon

Pinch nutmeg

DIRECTIONS

1 Preheat the oven to 400 degrees, and line a baking sheet with parchment paper.

2 Place the butternut squash cubes on the sheet and drizzle with oil.

3 Season with salt and pepper; then roast for 40 minutes or until tender.

4 Remove the squash from the oven and spoon into a blender.

5 Add the remaining ingredients and blend smooth.

6 Adjust the seasoning to taste, and serve hot.

PER SERVING: *Calories 126 (From Fat 76); Fat 9g (Saturated 5g); Cholesterol 0mg; Sodium 622mg; Carbohydrate 12g (Dietary Fiber 3g); Net Carbohydrate 9g; Protein 2g.*

Crispy Bacon Chicken and Garlic Spinach

| PREP TIME: 5 MIN | COOK TIME: 15 MIN | YIELD: 4 SERVINGS |

INGREDIENTS

4 slices bacon

8 bone-in chicken thighs

Salt and pepper, to taste

4 cloves garlic

¾ cup chicken broth

1 tablespoon unsalted butter

2 cups fresh baby spinach

DIRECTIONS

1 In a large cast-iron skillet, cook the bacon over medium-high heat until crisp.

2 Remove the bacon and drain some of the fat from the skillet. Crumble the bacon when cooled.

3 Reheat the bacon grease in the skillet over medium-high heat and add the chicken skin-side-down along with the diced garlic.

4 Cook for 6 to 8 minutes, until the skin is crisp; then flip and season with salt and pepper.

5 Let the chicken cook for another 8 minutes, until cooked through; then remove only the chicken to a plate.

6 Add the chicken broth to the skillet, scrape up any browned bits, and then add the butter.

7 Return the chicken to the skillet, and cook until the sauce starts to thicken.

8 Stir in the spinach and cook until the spinach is just wilted; then sprinkle with bacon to serve.

PER SERVING: *Calories 719 (From Fat 437); Fat 49g (Saturated 15g); Cholesterol 383mg; Sodium 713mg; Carbohydrate 3g (Dietary Fiber 1g); Net Carbohydrate 2g; Protein 65g.*

Sausage and Slaw Skillet

| PREP TIME: 5 MIN | COOK TIME: 20 MIN | YIELD: 4 SERVINGS |

INGREDIENTS

Six 3-ounce Italian sausage links

1 tablespoon olive oil

1 small yellow onion, diced

1 small red bell pepper, cored and diced

Salt and pepper, to taste

3 cloves minced garlic

½ teaspoon dried oregano

½ teaspoon paprika

Pinch red pepper flakes

2 cups shredded green cabbage

½ cup shredded red cabbage

1 cup sliced Brussels sprouts

½ cup finely chopped kale

DIRECTIONS

1 Place the sausages in a medium cast-iron skillet, and add enough water so they're mostly submerged.

2 Bring the water to a boil; then turn off the heat and let the sausages sit for 5 to 7 minutes, until cooked through.

3 Drain the water; then return the skillet to the heat and brown the sausages on all sides.

4 Remove the sausages to a cutting board, and slice when cool enough to handle.

5 Heat the oil in the same skillet on medium heat.

6 Add the onions and peppers and sauté for 2 to 3 minutes; then season with salt and pepper.

7 Add the garlic, oregano, paprika, and red pepper flakes, and cook for another 30 seconds.

8 Stir in the cabbage, Brussels sprouts, and kale; cook, stirring often, until it starts to wilt, about 4 to 6 minutes.

9 Adjust the seasoning to taste; then add the sliced sausages back to the skillet and cook until heated through. Serve hot.

PER SERVING: *Calories 293 (From Fat 193); Fat 22g (Saturated 7g); Cholesterol 37mg; Sodium 949mg; Carbohydrate 11g (Dietary Fiber 3g); Net Carbohydrate 8g; Protein 15g.*

Pan-Fried Pork Chops with Mushroom Gravy

PREP TIME: 5 MIN	COOK TIME: 15 MIN	YIELD: 4 SERVINGS

INGREDIENTS

Four 5-ounce boneless pork loin chops

1 teaspoon dried thyme

Salt and pepper, to taste

2 tablespoons unsalted butter, divided

1 pound sliced mushrooms

1 small yellow onion, dice

2 cloves minced garlic

½ cup white wine

¼ cup chicken broth

½ cup heavy cream

DIRECTIONS

1 Season the pork chops with thyme, salt, and pepper.

2 In a large skillet, heat half of the butter over medium-high heat, and add the pork chops.

3 Cook for 3 to 4 minutes per side, until browned; then remove to a plate and keep warm.

4 Reheat the skillet with the remaining butter and add the mushrooms; swirl to coat with butter.

5 Cook for 1 minute; then stir in the onions and garlic and cook for 2 minutes more.

6 Add the wine and chicken broth, scraping up the browned bits from the bottom of the pan.

7 Simmer on medium-low until reduced by half; then stir in the cream.

8 Simmer until the sauce is thickened; then add the pork chops back to the skillet.

9 Cook until the pork is just heated through; then serve with the mushroom gravy.

PER SERVING: *Calories 375 (From Fat 215); Fat 24g (Saturated 13g); Cholesterol 128mg; Sodium 182mg; Carbohydrate 8g (Dietary Fiber 2g); Net Carbohydrate 6g; Protein 32g.*

One-Pot Creamy Cauliflower Chowder

| PREP TIME: 20 MIN | COOK TIME: 45 MIN | YIELD: 4 SERVINGS |

INGREDIENTS

4 slices bacon, chopped

1 tablespoon unsalted butter

½ small yellow onion, diced

1 small carrot, diced

1 small stalk celery, diced

1 medium head cauliflower, chopped

2 cloves minced garlic

½ teaspoon dried thyme

2 cups vegetable broth

1½ cups heavy cream

Salt and pepper, to taste

DIRECTIONS

1 In a Dutch over, cook the bacon over medium-high heat until crisp.

2 With a slotted spoon, remove the bacon to a paper towel to drain.

3 Add the butter, onion, carrot, and celery and cook over medium-high heat for 2 minutes.

4 Stir in the cauliflower and cook on low heat for 12 to 15 minutes, until tender.

5 Stir in the garlic and thyme, and cook for 1 minute more.

6 Pour in the broth and heavy cream, and season with salt and pepper.

7 Simmer for 30 minutes on low heat; then garnish with bacon bits to serve.

PER SERVING: Calories 455 (From Fat 375); Fat 42g (Saturated 25g); Cholesterol 142mg; Sodium 858mg; Carbohydrate 15g (Dietary Fiber 4g); Net Carbohydrate 11g; Protein 8g.

Hearty Vegetable Soup

INGREDIENTS

1 tablespoon olive oil

½ small yellow onion, diced

1 small red pepper, diced

2 cloves minced garlic

1½ cups chopped cauliflower

1 cup sliced green beans

½ cup diced tomatoes

2½ cups chicken broth

1 teaspoon dried Italian seasoning

1 small bay leaf

Salt and pepper, to taste

Fresh chopped parsley

DIRECTIONS

1 In a large saucepan, heat the oil over medium heat.

2 Add the onions and peppers, and sauté for 6 to 8 minutes, until browned.

3 Stir in the garlic, and sauté for 1 minute.

4 Add the cauliflower, green beans, tomatoes, broth, Italian seasoning, bay leaf, salt, and pepper.

5 Bring to a boil; then reduce the heat and simmer on low, covered, for 15 minutes, until the vegetables are tender.

6 Garnish with fresh chopped parsley.

PER SERVING: *Calories 75 (From Fat 39); Fat 4g (Saturated 1g); Cholesterol 0mg; Sodium 735mg; Carbohydrate 8g (Dietary Fiber 3g); Net Carbohydrate 5g; Protein 3g.*

Meaty Skillet Lasagna with Zucchini Noodles

INGREDIENTS

2 medium zucchini

1 teaspoon olive oil

12 ounces 80 percent lean ground beef

1 cup diced mushrooms

2 cloves minced garlic

Salt and pepper, to taste

3 tablespoons tomato paste

1 cup diced tomatoes

1 cup no-sugar-added marinara sauce

1 teaspoon dried oregano

1 teaspoon dried basil

1½ cups shredded mozzarella cheese

¼ cup full-fat ricotta cheese

Dried parsley, to serve

DIRECTIONS

1 Use a vegetable peeler to peel the zucchini into wide noodles; pat dry with paper towel.

2 In a large skillet, heat the oil on medium–high heat, and add the beef.

3 Cook until browned, about 4 to 5 minutes, breaking it up with a wooden spoon.

4 Drain the excess fat; then stir in the mushrooms and garlic; season with salt and pepper.

5 Stir in the tomato paste, tomatoes, marinara sauce, oregano, and basil; then bring to a boil.

6 Reduce the heat and simmer for 5 minutes; then stir in the zucchini noodles and cover.

7 Cook for 3 to 4 minutes; then remove from heat and stir in the mozzarella cheese.

8 Adjust the seasoning to taste, and top with dollops of ricotta cheese and dried parsley to serve.

PER SERVING: *Calories 375 (From Fat 199); Fat 22g (Saturated 11g); Cholesterol 93mg; Sodium 895mg; Carbohydrate 15g (Dietary Fiber 4g); Net Carbohydrate 11g; Protein 29g.*

Chapter **20**

Desserts: Having Your Sweets and Eating Them, Too

Because carbohydrates turn into sugar, many new low-carb dieters struggle with sweet-tooth cravings in the first three weeks as they transition into ketosis. Depending on what your sugar intake looked like before launching your keto journey, this could be a pretty significant testing ground for self-control and sticking to your meal plan and macros.

The good news is that you don't have to avoid sweets — you just have to be very intentional about how you approach them and which recipes you use. With natural sweeteners that are actually healthy — such as stevia, monk fruit, and erythritol — now readily available, you can easily adapt a number of recipes to fit your requirements on the ketogenic diet.

We've found that uncontrolled cravings can wreck your diet more easily than nearly anything else. You'll always need to have an element of self-control, of course, but our entire mission in the keto world centers around giving you access to the most delicious foods available without sacrificing quality by going low-carb. If we can possibly make a keto-friendly version of something, we're all over it.

This can also be a great "keto evangelism" tool. There are few things more mind-blowing to people who oppose keto than to challenge their assumptions about treats being out of the game by showing up to a party with a sinfully delicious, low-carb dessert in hand. Many opponents of keto paint the diet as something that's boring, tasteless, and devoid of anything that resembles sweetness.

In this chapter, we give you some great options to introduce you to the world of delectable, healthy desserts that your friends likely won't be able to tell from the real thing. Each recipe requires a maximum combined prep and cook time of less than 30 minutes, with ingredients and directions that are easy to find, simple to follow, and mind-blowing to eat.

Strawberries and Cream Pancakes

PREP TIME: 10 MIN	COOK TIME: 15 MIN	YIELD: 2 SERVINGS

INGREDIENTS

2 large eggs, separated

½ teaspoon cream of tartar

2 ounces chopped cream cheese, divided

½ teaspoon vanilla extract

¼ teaspoon ground cinnamon

8 to 12 drops liquid stevia extract, to taste

½ cup sliced strawberries

1 teaspoon olive oil

¼ cup sugar-free whipped cream

DIRECTIONS

1 In a medium bowl, beat the egg whites with a hand mixer until foamy, about 30 seconds.

2 Add the cream of tartar and beat on high speed until stiff peaks form.

3 In a separate bowl, beat together the egg yolks, cream cheese, vanilla extract, cinnamon, and stevia until well combined.

4 Fold in the egg whites and strawberries.

5 Spoon the batter onto a greased and preheated griddle using ¼ cup per pancake, and cook on low heat for 4 to 5 minutes until nearly cooked through.

6 Carefully flip the pancakes and cook until browned underneath, about 1 to 2 minutes.

7 Slide the pancakes onto a plate and keep warm while you prepare the rest of the pancakes.

8 Serve warm with whipped cream on top.

PER SERVING: Calories 259 (From Fat 201); Fat 22g (Saturated 11g); Cholesterol 238mg; Sodium 169mg; Carbohydrate 6g (Dietary Fiber 1g); Net Carbohydrate 5g; Protein 9g.

Easy Cinnamon Mug Cake

PREP TIME: 5 MIN | **COOK TIME: 10 MIN** | **YIELD: 1 SERVING**

INGREDIENTS

2 tablespoons powdered erythritol, divided

¾ teaspoon ground cinnamon, divided

¼ cup almond flour

¼ teaspoon ground nutmeg

Pinch salt

1 large egg

1 tablespoon unsalted butter, melted

½ teaspoon vanilla extract

Sugar-free maple syrup

DIRECTIONS

1 In a small bowl, combine ½ tablespoon of the erythritol with ¼ teaspoon of the cinnamon; set aside.

2 Preheat the oven to 350 degrees, and grease a 4-ounce ramekin with cooking spray.

3 In a small bowl, whisk together the almond flour with the remaining erythritol, the remaining cinnamon, the nutmeg, and the salt until well combined.

4 Stir in the egg, butter, and vanilla extract until smooth.

5 Pour the mixture into the greased ramekin and sprinkle on the erythritol and cinnamon mixture.

6 Bake for 12 minutes (or microwave on high for 1 minute) until set.

7 Drizzle with sugar-free maple syrup and serve in the ramekin.

PER SERVING: *Calories 349 (From Fat 273); Fat 31g (Saturated 10g); Cholesterol 217mg; Sodium 236mg; Carbohydrate 11g (Dietary Fiber 4g); Net Carbohydrate 7g; Protein 13g.*

Creamy Cookie Dough Mousse

PREP TIME: 10 MIN | COOK TIME: 3 MIN | YIELD: 2 SERVINGS

INGREDIENTS

2 tablespoons unsalted butter

4 ounces cream cheese, softened

¼ cup powdered erythritol

1 teaspoon sugar-free maple syrup

1½ teaspoons vanilla extract

¼ cup stevia-sweetened dark chocolate chips

DIRECTIONS

1 In a small saucepan, melt the butter over low heat until golden brown.

2 In a medium bowl, beat together the cream cheese, erythritol, maple syrup, and vanilla extract with a hand mixer until smooth and well combined.

3 Beat in the browned butter until smooth and well combined.

4 Fold in the chocolate chips; then spoon into two dessert cups and chill until ready to serve.

PER SERVING: *Calories 378 (From Fat 334); Fat 37g (Saturated 22g); Cholesterol 93mg; Sodium 184mg; Carbohydrate 16g (Dietary Fiber 6g); Net Carbohydrate 10g; Protein 5g.*

TIP: If you're looking for dark chocolate chips, Lily's is a great brand to try.

Pumpkin Pudding

INGREDIENTS

½ cup canned coconut milk

¼ cup powdered erythritol

3 tablespoons canned pumpkin puree

1 teaspoon vanilla extract

1 teaspoon pumpkin pie spice

⅛ teaspoon xanthan gum

2 tablespoons whipped cream

Pinch ground cinnamon

DIRECTIONS

1 In a medium saucepan, whisk together the coconut milk, erythritol, pumpkin, vanilla, pumpkin pie spice, and xanthan gum over medium heat.

2 Whisk continuously for 1 minute.

3 Spoon into a bowl and chill for 30 minutes until set.

4 Divide among small bowls and top with whipped cream and cinnamon to serve.

PER SERVING: *Calories 133 (From Fat 108); Fat 12g (Saturated 11g); Cholesterol 10mg; Sodium 20mg; Carbohydrate 4g (Dietary Fiber 1g); Net Carbohydrate 3g; Protein 2g.*

Lemon Jell-O Cake

PREP TIME: 15 MIN	COOK TIME: 15 MIN	YIELD: 4 SERVINGS

INGREDIENTS

1 cup unsalted pecans

1 teaspoon monk fruit and erythritol blend sweetener, 1:1 sweetness of sugar

½ teaspoon ground cinnamon

Pinch salt

1 tablespoon unsalted butter, melted

One 0.3-ounce packet sugar-free lemon Jell-O powder

⅔ cup boiling water

One 8-ounce package cream cheese, softened

2 tablespoons fresh lemon juice

1 teaspoon fresh lemon zest

DIRECTIONS

1 Preheat the oven to 350 degrees and grease a 6-x-6-inch baking dish with butter.

2 Place the pecans, monk fruit erythritol sweetener, cinnamon, and salt in a food processor.

3 Pulse the mixture until it forms a crumblike texture; then pulse in the melted butter until it comes together.

4 Press the mixture into the prepared baking dish.

5 Bake for 12 to 15 minutes until dry to the touch and just browned; then cool for 15 minutes.

6 In a medium bowl, combine the Jell-O powder with the boiling water and stir until it dissolves.

7 Add the cream cheese, lemon juice, and lemon zest, and then stir until smooth.

8 Pour the mixture into the crust and chill overnight until set; cut into 4 squares to serve.

PER SERVING: *Calories 404 (From Fat 361); Fat 40g (Saturated 14g); Cholesterol 70mg; Sodium 276mg; Carbohydrate 7g (Dietary Fiber 3g); Net Carbohydrate 4g; Protein 7g.*

Key Lime Panna Cotta

| PREP TIME: 10 MIN | COOK TIME: 2 MIN | YIELD: 4 SERVINGS |

INGREDIENTS

2 cups heavy cream

One 8-gram packet unflavored gelatin

¼ cup granulated erythritol

4 key limes, juiced and zested

½ teaspoon vanilla extract

Pinch salt

1 tablespoon coconut oil

¼ cup almond flour

1 teaspoon granulated erythritol

Pinch ground cinnamon

DIRECTIONS

1 In a medium saucepan, whisk together the heavy cream, gelatin, and ¼ cup erythritol over medium–low heat.

2 Stir until the erythritol dissolves; then whisk in the lime juice, lime zest, vanilla extract, and salt.

3 Grease four small ramekins with coconut oil; then pour the panna cotta batter into them.

4 Chill for 4 to 6 hours up to overnight until set.

5 Before serving, combine the almond flour, erythritol, and cinnamon in a small bowl.

6 Add the mixture to a warm skillet and cook over low heat until just toasted.

7 Sprinkle the panna cotta with the toasted mixture to serve.

PER SERVING: *Calories 512 (From Fat 460); Fat 51g (Saturated 31g); Cholesterol 164mg; Sodium 87mg; Carbohydrate 12g (Dietary Fiber 3g); Net Carbohydrate 9g; Protein 6g.*

Banana Almond Muffins

PREP TIME: 10 MIN | COOK TIME: 18 MIN | YIELD: 6 MUFFINS

INGREDIENTS

1 cup almond butter

⅔ cup powdered erythritol

3 large eggs

1½ teaspoons vanilla extract

1 teaspoon baking powder

½ teaspoon banana extract

Pinch salt

¼ cup slivered almonds

DIRECTIONS

1 Preheat the oven to 325 degrees, and line half a muffin pan with paper liners.

2 In a blender, combine the almond butter and erythritol and blend until smooth.

3 Add the eggs, vanilla, baking powder, banana extract, and salt, and blend again until smooth.

4 Divide among the 6 muffin cups.

5 Sprinkle with almonds and bake for 16 to 18 minutes, until set.

PER SERVING: *Calories 292 (From Fat 221); Fat 25g (Saturated 2g); Cholesterol 93mg; Sodium 126mg; Carbohydrate 8g (Dietary Fiber 6g); Net Carbohydrate 2g; Protein 13g.*

Mint Chocolate Chip Ice Cream

INGREDIENTS

2 cups canned coconut milk, unsweetened

¼ cup heavy cream

¾ cup powdered erythritol

1 medium avocado, pitted and chopped

1 teaspoon vanilla extract

½ teaspoon mint extract

½ cup stevia-sweetened dark chocolate chips

DIRECTIONS

1 Freeze the ice cream maker's drum overnight or according to the manufacturer's instructions.

2 In a food processor, combine the coconut milk, cream, erythritol, avocado, vanilla extract, and mint extract and blend until smooth and well combined.

3 Pour the mixture into the frozen ice cream drum and churn it according to the manufacturer's instructions.

4 Spoon the mixture into an airtight container, fold in the chocolate chips quickly, and freeze overnight.

5 Thaw the ice cream for 10 to 15 minutes at room temperature before scooping to serve.

PER SERVING: *Calories 187 (From Fat 162); Fat 18g (Saturated 13g); Cholesterol 10mg; Sodium 18mg; Carbohydrate 10g (Dietary Fiber 4g); Net Carbohydrate 6g; Protein 3g.*

TIP: If you're looking for dark chocolate chips, Lily's is a great brand to try.

Avocado Chocolate Mousse

PREP TIME: 10 MIN	COOK TIME: NONE	YIELD: 4 SERVINGS

INGREDIENTS

½ teaspoon instant coffee powder

2 tablespoons heavy cream

2 medium avocados

2 tablespoons unsweetened cocoa powder

3 tablespoons powdered erythritol

1 teaspoon vanilla extract

¼ cup whipped cream

DIRECTIONS

1 Dissolve the coffee powder into the heavy cream.

2 Peel the avocados and remove the pits.

3 Scoop the avocado flesh into a blender and add the dissolved coffee power, cream, cocoa powder, erythritol, and vanilla extract.

4 Blend until smooth and creamy.

5 Spoon into dessert cups and top with whipped cream to serve.

PER SERVING: *Calories 186 (From Fat 155); Fat 17g (Saturated 5g); Cholesterol 21mg; Sodium 6mg; Carbohydrate 10g (Dietary Fiber 3g); Net Carbohydrate 7g; Protein 3g.*

Almond Fudge Brownies

PREP TIME: 15 MIN | COOK TIME: 12 MIN | YIELD: 12 BROWNIES

INGREDIENTS

1 cup almond butter

¾ cup powdered erythritol

10 tablespoons unsweetened cocoa powder

3 large eggs

1 teaspoon vanilla extract

½ teaspoon baking powder

¼ cup stevia-sweetened dark chocolate chips

DIRECTIONS

1 Preheat the oven to 325 degrees and grease a 9-x-9-inch baking dish with cooking spray.

2 In a food processor, combine the almond butter and erythritol and blend until smooth.

3 Add the cocoa powder, eggs, vanilla, and baking powder to the blender.

4 Pulse several times and then blend until smooth.

5 Spread the batter in the prepared pan and sprinkle with dark chocolate chips.

6 Bake for 10 to 12 minutes, until set; then cool completely before slicing to serve.

PER SERVING: *Calories 155 (From Fat 115); Fat 13g (Saturated 2g); Cholesterol 47mg; Sodium 35mg; Carbohydrate 8g (Dietary Fiber 5g); Net Carbohydrate 3g; Protein 7g.*

TIP: If you're looking for dark chocolate chips, Lily's is a great brand to try.

Banana Pudding

PREP TIME: 10 MIN	COOK TIME: 5 MIN	YIELD: 1 SERVING

INGREDIENTS

½ cup heavy cream

3 tablespoons powdered erythritol

1 large egg yolk

1 teaspoon vanilla extract

½ teaspoon xanthan gum

½ teaspoon banana extract

Pinch salt

¼ cup sugar-free whipped cream

DIRECTIONS

1 In a double boiler, combine the cream, erythritol, and egg yolk over medium-low heat.

2 Whisk constantly until the erythritol dissolves and the mixture thickens.

3 Stir in the vanilla and xanthan gum and whisk for 1 minute more.

4 Add the banana extract and salt; stir until well combined.

5 Spoon into a small dish and cover with plastic, the film touching the pudding.

6 Chill for 4 hours; then spoon into dessert cups.

7 Top with whipped cream to serve.

PER SERVING: *Calories 592 (From Fat 540); Fat 60g (Saturated 36g); Cholesterol 390mg; Sodium 67mg; Carbohydrate 7g (Dietary Fiber 1g); Net Carbohydrate 6g; Protein 6g.*

6

The Part of Tens

Discover ten benefits of low-carb living.

Read about the best healthy fats.

Find the most helpful keto resources.

Chapter **21**

Ten Benefits of Being in Ketosis

I n this chapter, we give you a quick look at our top ten reasons for sticking to keto and how it will change your life for the better.

Jump-Starting Weight Loss

The verdict is in: If you've tried every diet under the sun and you haven't been able to lose weight or, worse, you've regained all the weight you lost and more, the keto diet may be the answer you've been looking for. Research has consistently shown that people on the keto diet lose more weight and keep it off longer than people on low-fat, high-carb diets.

Stabilizing Blood Sugar

Diabetes is rampant in western society. Up to one-third of Americans are prediabetic, and many don't even know it. Keto is a safe and natural way to make sure your blood sugars are always in a healthy and normal range. With normal blood sugar levels, you won't have high levels of insulin, the hormone that over time causes you to pack on pounds and leads to diabetes if levels get too high. The keto diet is so effective that some doctors and nutritionists recommend the keto diet to manage and even reverse type 2 diabetes!

Increasing Energy

Ketosis is a fuel-efficient way for the body — and the brain — to run on fats. Many people on the keto diet notice more energy and a general joie de vivre that they've been missing on a high-carb diet. You experience no sugar swings or carb cravings. Instead, you're letting your body do what it does best: Thrive.

Lowering Cholesterol Levels

Fat is good for you! Studies show that the range of fats in a well-rounded keto diet helps to improve your cholesterol numbers by

>> Decreasing triglyceride levels

>> Decreasing low-density lipoprotein (LDL), or "bad" cholesterol

>> Increasing high-density lipoprotein (HDL), or "good" cholesterol

Improving your cholesterol numbers is critical to keeping your heart healthy and preventing cardiovascular disease like heart attack and stroke.

Lowering Blood Pressure

High blood pressure is another common ailment that plagues a lot of Americans. High blood pressure is known as the "silent killer" because most people who have it have no idea they're affected. A low-carbohydrate diet has been shown to lower blood pressure, and the complications that come along with it, so you won't have anything to worry about and can expect a long and healthy life.

Getting Better Sleep

The keto diet is an excellent tool for getting those much needed zzz's. It increases the amount of time you spend in the most regenerative parts of sleep — deep sleep and rapid eye movement (REM) sleep. You'll get more restful sleep even when you can't get as many hours as you'd like. That means no wasted time counting sheep or staring at the clock.

Eliminating Cravings

Eating a high-fat, low-carb diet naturally shuts down pesky sugar cravings. Without the drug-like addiction to carbs, you'll experience freedom like never before.

High-fat foods leave you feeling satisfied, energetic, and with no thoughts of your next meal. Without thoughts of dinner or cake — or regrets about overindulging weighing heavily on your mind — you'll be energized to focus on the things you love and care about.

Looking Your Best

Not only does sugar cause cravings and weight gain, but it's also a trigger for acne. If you're looking for a safe and natural treatment for facial acne, the keto diet may be the answer you've been looking for.

Some dermatologists are now recommending low-carb diets to teenagers and others who can't get rid of acne despite trying a host of prescription medicines. So, the keto lifestyle not only keeps you healthy, but also keeps you looking good as well!

Lifting Your Mood

Most people on the keto journey notice that the little things don't phase them as much as they used to when they ate bread and pasta regularly. That's because, unlike carbs, which contribute to brain fog, ketosis increases

>> **Ketones,** which decrease inflammation and strengthen the connection between brain cells

>> **Substances like adenosine and gamma aminobutyric acid (GABA),** which calm your brain cells and limit overexciting brain cells

Continuing the keto lifestyle may help you shake off the blues and see the sunnier aspects of life.

Stopping Inflammation in Its Tracks

Many of the chronic illnesses that plague Americans are a result of inflammation that is a direct result of overindulgence in sugars and other high-carb foods. The keto diet works hard to keep your body healthy and inflammation-free, which prevents things like heart disease, cancer, fibromyalgia, and a host of other conditions.

Chapter 22

Ten Sources of Healthy Fats

Not all fats are created equal. The benefits of ketosis come from its focus on getting the majority of your calories from high-quality fats. In this chapter, we give you our ten favorite fats that keep us healthy, full, and loving the keto lifestyle.

Avocado/Avocado Oil

The mighty avocado is a keto dieter's dream food. Filled with hearth healthy monounsaturated fatty acids (MUFAs), avocados are packed with vitamins and minerals like potassium and magnesium to help you get through the keto flu (see Chapter 2). What's more, these keto-friendly fruits are also good sources of fiber and antioxidants, which help contribute to keto's overall anti-inflammatory mode of operation. Avocados have a great, creamy texture that's perfect in smoothies and desserts, as well as in salads and soups. With the avocado, the options are endless!

Ghee

Ghee, a type of butter that has been heated to remove milk fats and water, is a denser, healthier version of butter. It has fat-soluble vitamins and has been used for thousands of years in *Ayurveda* (a form of traditional Indian healing) to help decrease inflammation and promote health. Research shows that Ayurvedic doctors had it right: The short- and medium-chain fatty acids in ghee are associated with fat loss and heart health, as well as improved digestion and gut health.

When choosing ghee, and any other dairy product, make sure it comes from grass-fed cows. Ghee is excellent for sautéing veggies and grilling proteins. It adds a nutty flavor to your food.

Coconut Oil

Coconut oil is high in saturated fat, but unlike animal-based saturated fats, it's about 50 percent medium-chain fats that our bodies tend to turn into fat-burning fuel quickly. Studies show that coconut oil improves high-density lipoprotein (HDL) levels and helps fight bacteria that cause infections. Like ghee, coconut oil is great for grilling and frying and adds flavor to your foods.

Olive Oil

The powerhouse of the Mediterranean diet, olive oil is known for its heart-healthy MUFAs. Olive oil helps to decrease blood pressure and reduces your risk of heart attack and stroke, while helping you maintain a healthy weight. Plus, it contains a whopping 75 percent of your daily value of both vitamins E and K. Olive oil is chock-full of antioxidants that may help decrease your risk of inflammatory disease like Alzheimer's.

Choose extra virgin oil, which retains more of its antioxidants and isn't made with harmful chemicals like refined versions of olive oil. Like coconut oil and ghee, olive oil is excellent for cooking, but it's also great to use at room temperature (for example, as a base for your salad dressing).

Almonds

Nuts are an excellent multifunctional keto food, whether eaten raw, roasted, or lightly salted. In addition to consisting of 65 percent MUFAs, almonds are high in magnesium and manganese, as well as being a good source of anti-inflammatory antioxidants like vitamin E. Almonds are great as snacks, added to salads and soups, or pulverized to make a keto-friendly flour. Plus, almonds are a low-carb, moderate protein, and high-fat food (exactly like keto overall) and will keep you satisfied while you're on the run. There's no reason not to reach for a handful of almonds!

Grass-Fed Beef

Like almonds, meat is an excellent source of fat and protein that's very satisfying. However, not all beef is the same. Cows who roam freely and eat grass, rather than processed corn (which is the typical feed for factory-made beef), produce more omega-3s, beta-carotene, vitamin E, and MUFAs, significantly improving the quality of their meat. Besides, grass-fed beef is usually organic, meaning the cows aren't fed harmful antibiotics or hormones to increase their yield.

TIP

Grass-fed beef may be more expensive and harder to find, but it's worth the cost and effort. Find a local farmer's market if grocery stores near you don't carry grass-fed beef.

Medium-Chain Triglyceride Oils

Medium-chain triglyceride (MCT) oils are the basis for most of coconut oil's many benefits. Medium-chain fats are easier to digest than other types of saturated fat and are burned more quickly as fuel. MCT oils help improve your cholesterol levels and may help block the rise of *ghrelin* (the appetite-stimulating hormone that typically rises in people who go on diets). Also, MCT oils help combat constipation and are a great way to kick-start ketosis.

TIP

MCT oil is a useful supplement to help get back in ketosis for those who choose the cyclical ketogenic diet (see Chapter 1). Remember, however, that your digestive system needs to adapt to significant dietary changes, and overloading your system with MCTs may cause an upset stomach or diarrhea. Gradually incorporate more healthy oils into your diet, and you'll be fine.

Fatty Fish

Fatty fish includes great options like mackerel, salmon, trout, and canned varieties like sardines and anchovies. Oily fish are known for heart health benefits because of their high levels of omega-3 fatty acids. They're also excellent sources of fat-soluble vitamins like vitamin D, and studies show that people who eat higher amounts of fish tend to have a lower rate of age-related memory problems. Some people are concerned about eating fish because of high mercury levels, but fatty fish are generally low in that toxin.

WARNING

Although fish is tremendously healthy, there are some health risks that come with consuming too much. Many saltwater fish contain traces of mercury, which is fine in minute amounts because your body can flush it out of its system. Over a long time, however, eating large amounts of fish can cause mercury to slowly build up in your system until it reaches toxic levels. Experts recommend that you limit your weekly fish consumption to 8 to 12 ounces to avoid any potential complications.

Hemp Seeds

Hemp seeds are a great addition to a keto-friendly diet. These nuts from the hemp plant — with little to none of the active substance in marijuana — have a higher protein content than either chia seeds or flaxseeds. In addition to the fat, they're also rich in many minerals, such as zinc and magnesium, that are important to the keto lifestyle. Like ghee in India, hemp seeds have also been used for thousands of years in traditional Chinese medicine, and for good reason. Studies show that nutrients found in them help decrease heart disease. Hemp seeds can be added to salads or keto-friendly desserts or just eaten as an on-the-go snack.

Nut Butters

Like nuts, nut butters are a great addition to the keto diet. They're an excellent dip for your low-carb veggies, and they can be used to make a high-fat, moderate-protein marinade or as an alternate ingredient for keto desserts. When you're shopping, pay attention to the labels, and only purchase options that have peanuts and salt as ingredients; many common brands include partially hydrogenated oils and copious amounts of sugar, although plenty of all-natural options exist.

TIP

Make sure to choose options like almond butter, tahini, or peanut butter due to their low carb content. Some nut butters (and nuts) are higher in carbs than others — for example, both almond butter and peanut butter have fewer carbs per serving than cashew butter.

Chapter **23**

Ten Keto Resources

One of the most important ingredients to successful dieting is making sure that you're referencing the right resources. Getting high-quality information from qualified authorities is just as important as getting top-shelf ingredients for cooking.

Studies have repeatedly shown that partnering with another person or a community that's committed to the same goals you have is a critical factor in maintaining steady weight loss, as well as keeping it off when you're done!

In this chapter, we list what we consider the top ten keto resources, including keto communities. In addition to providing excellent information, these websites are filled with outstanding, supportive people who are committed to living their best low-carb lives.

Diet Doctor

One of the most qualified low-carb sources on the Internet, Diet Doctor (www.dietdoctor.com) provides a host of information in the form of keto guides, recipes, health information, videos, and news. Each of the Diet Doctor guides is either written or reviewed by medical doctors before it's published, so you know that you're getting the most accurate data possible.

Total Keto Diet App

We developed the Total Keto Diet app (www.totalketodiet.com) to be a one-stop shop for the low-carb dieter. Keeping track of your macros, and then translating those into recipes, only to have to convert them again into a grocery list — well, let's just say the complication adds up quickly. This app gives you access to hundreds of recipes with nutrition information already calculated, including calories and macros. You can instantly add the ingredients to an in-app grocery list, making meal selection, macro calculation, and shopping tasks you can accomplish without ever leaving the app. Bonus features include a meal-planning service, keto news section, and macros calculator.

Healthline Nutrition

Healthline Nutrition (www.healthline.com/nutrition) is an outstanding source of information for every aspect of low-carb dieting. Not only does it provide one of the most comprehensive libraries of keto data available, but each article is written and fact-checked by licensed nutritionists and dietitians before publication.

The information you'll find here goes far beyond typical "eat this, don't eat that" diet advice. You can find articles discussing how collagen affects your hair health or how lowering your carbohydrate intake can benefit your skin. If you have a question about how the ketogenic diet will affect your life, start here.

Tasteaholics

We started Tasteaholics (www.tasteaholics.com) after we fell in love with keto. We let our own journey drive the content, constantly asking ourselves, "What would we have liked to have as a resource when we first got started?"

After many years of experience, we deeply understand all the hardships of starting or getting back into the keto diet. That's why you'll find hundreds of low-carb recipes and dozens of science-backed articles about the keto diet and other health topics.

Peter Attia

A licensed medical doctor, Peter Attia (www.peterattiamd.com) is one of the most innovative thinkers in the low-carb world. His articles, podcasts, videos, and interview series are incredibly informative. Dr. Attia was one of the primary motivating factors when we first decided to try the ketogenic diet, and the information he publishes is so informative that we still visit his site regularly and come away with a new revelation every time.

TIP

Check out his talk on YouTube called "An Advantaged Metabolic State: Human Performance, Resilience & Health" (https://youtu.be/NqwvcrA7oe8). It's one of the first things we watched about the keto diet, and it started us down this incredible keto diet rabbit hole.

Mark's Daily Apple

Mark Sisson, the creator of the Primal Blueprint series (www.marksdailyapple.com/primal-blueprint-101). He focuses on taking the best and forgotten parts of our ancestral traditions and combining them with modern living to allow us to genuinely live the best possible life. His website, Mark's Daily Apple (www.marksdailyapple.com), is filled with resources, from recipes to fitness routines. If you're looking for a lifestyle that goes beyond simple weight loss, we're sure you'll be intrigued by what Mark has to offer.

KetoConnect

If you want to find out more about keto in a way that's customized to your favorite method of ingesting information, check out KetoConnect (www.ketoconnect.net). This site publishes resources on every major social media platform, including YouTube. It also features an informative podcast (www.ketoconnect.net/keto-for-normies), along with tons of meal-planning and meal-prepping resources. You can find a host of interactive programs here as well.

Reddit's /r/keto Subreddit

Arguably the largest keto-focused group on the planet, the /r/keto subreddit (www.reddit.com/r/keto) offers a wealth of interactive information. With more than 1 million subscribers, thousands of members are online at any given time. If you're struggling with a keto issue that's specific to you and you can't seem to find the answer, drop a line here. You're almost guaranteed to find a number of fellow dieters who've wrestled with — and overcome — the exact same problem.

Keto Macro Calculator

Although Tasteaholics has its own keto macro calculator (`www.tasteaholics.com/keto-calculator`), you'll find various other calculators at quality sites across the Internet. This will always be your starting point on keto, because your macros determine everything. Here are two we recommend:

>> `www.perfectketo.com/keto-macro-calculator`

>> `www.wholesomeyum.com/the-best-free-low-carb-keto-macro-calculator`

Because all calculators run macros slightly differently, the best approach is to use two or three and average your results.

REMEMBER

If you run your numbers through more than one calculator, the results from each may vary slightly. Don't worry too much about this discrepancy — each calculator takes a slightly different approach, weighing options like job activity and fitness levels a bit differently. Visit several, average the numbers, and then take off. As you find what works best in your life, you'll be able to customize your macros to find what suits you best.

Facebook Keto and Low-Carb Groups

While the majority of the resources listed in this chapter are informative, nothing beats the support you get from interacting with peers who are on the same journey. Facebook is an excellent place to go for this, with groups both large and small to offer advice, feedback, and encouragement at every step.

Our Facebook group, Total Keto Diet (`www.facebook.com/groups/totalketodiet`), is a home for recipe sharing, success stories, and inspiration. Whether you've just started the low-carb lifestyle or you're a seasoned pro, there's something for you here. You can also find smaller groups that are specifically targeted to a specific geographic location or that focus on individual issues, such as PCOS or diabetes.

REMEMBER

You don't have to go this alone, and there are literally millions of people out there who want to help!

Metric Conversion Guide

Note: The recipes in this book weren't developed or tested using metric measurements. There may be some variation in quality when converting to metric units.

Common Abbreviations

Abbreviation(s)	What It Stands For
cm	Centimeter
C., c.	Cup
G, g	Gram
kg	Kilogram
L, l	Liter
lb.	Pound
mL, ml	Milliliter
oz.	Ounce
pt.	Pint
t., tsp.	Teaspoon
T., Tb., Tbsp.	Tablespoon

Volume

U.S. Units	Canadian Metric	Australian Metric
¼ teaspoon	1 milliliter	1 milliliter
½ teaspoon	2 milliliters	2 milliliters
1 teaspoon	5 milliliters	5 milliliters
1 tablespoon	15 milliliters	20 milliliters
¼ cup	50 milliliters	60 milliliters
⅓ cup	75 milliliters	80 milliliters

(continued)

(continued)

U.S. Units	Canadian Metric	Australian Metric
½ cup	125 milliliters	125 milliliters
⅔ cup	150 milliliters	170 milliliters
¾ cup	175 milliliters	190 milliliters
1 cup	250 milliliters	250 milliliters
1 quart	1 liter	1 liter
1½ quarts	1.5 liters	1.5 liters
2 quarts	2 liters	2 liters
2½ quarts	2.5 liters	2.5 liters
3 quarts	3 liters	3 liters
4 quarts (1 gallon)	4 liters	4 liters

Weight

U.S. Units	Canadian Metric	Australian Metric
1 ounce	30 grams	30 grams
2 ounces	55 grams	60 grams
3 ounces	85 grams	90 grams
4 ounces (¼ pound)	115 grams	125 grams
8 ounces (½ pound)	225 grams	225 grams
16 ounces (1 pound)	455 grams	500 grams (½ kilogram)

Length

Inches	Centimeters
0.5	1.5
1	2.5
2	5.0
3	7.5
4	10.0

Temperature (Degrees)

Fahrenheit	Celsius
32	0
212	100
250	120
275	140
300	150
325	160
350	180
375	190
400	200
425	220
450	230
475	240
500	260

Inches	Centimeters
5	12.5
6	15.0
7	17.5
8	20.5
9	23.0
10	25.5
11	28.0
12	30.5

Index

Symbols and Numerics

A

B

M

About the Authors

Rami Abrams and Vicky Abrams are two entrepreneurs based in Brooklyn, New York. They first discovered the keto diet in 2014 and were initially (and understandably) a little skeptical about a diet that allowed more butter and bacon intake than it did whole grains. Never ones to live with unsatisfied curiosity, they dug deep into the diet's backgrounds. They were impressed by its foundation as a peer-reviewed medical treatment and weight loss tool and decided to give it a shot. Within just a few weeks, they were steadily moving toward their goal weights and had never felt better in their lives.

Seeing the scale move in the right direction, seemingly effortlessly, was great, but the two biggest advantages they noticed were a steady energy state and increased mental clarity throughout the day. The further they traveled on their keto journey, the more consistent and energetic they felt; what started as a short-term experiment turned into a complete life transformation.

Both Rami and Vicky are self-professed "foodies" who love to try new dishes and genres at every opportunity. Although enthralled with their new way of "fat-focused" cooking with all the flavors it provided, the couple found that they were missing many of their old favorites. Determined to have their cake and eat it, too, they began to seek out new ways of re-creating established conventions in the kitchen.

It involved a few trials and errors (and several unfortunate encounters with the smoke detector), but eventually, they experienced a breakthrough. Vicky is fond of saying that there are ways of re-creating almost all your favorite foods, including dessert. For a diet that revolves around eliminating sugar and other harmful sweeteners, that's quite an achievement!

At the beginning of 2015, Rami and Vicky developed Tasteaholics.com and focused on writing research-heavy articles while also developing and photographing recipes and blogging about their progress. The site rapidly became renowned as an expert source for both keto information and tantalizing recipes. By the second year, they began publishing their popular series of cookbooks called *Keto in Five.* The cookbooks center on three basic principles: Every dish contains five or fewer grams of net carbs per serving, is made with up to five ingredients, and can be prepared in five easy steps. Their efforts were so successful that they were able to quit their jobs and focus exclusively on Tasteaholics.

In 2017, the Abrams launched So Nourished, Inc., a company dedicated to creating low-carb ingredients and products, such as healthy sugar replacements and low-carb brownies, pancake mixes, and syrups. They also expanded their sites to include meal plans and keto news articles and launched the Total Keto Diet mobile app.

Although they stay busy, the Abrams found plenty of time to engage in two of their favorite activities: traveling and trying new food. In one year, they spent six months exploring eight different countries, sampling each area's delicacies and blogging about the keto lifestyle and low-carb recipes from around the globe. As the healthy fat revolution continues, Rami and Vicky remain dedicated to spreading the word about the benefits of ketosis in every area of life.